THE ORGANIC FOOD GUIDE

HOW TO SHOP SMARTER AND EAT HEALTHIER

THE ORGANIC FOOD GUIDE

HOW TO SHOP SMARTER AND EAT HEALTHIER

Steve Meyerowitz

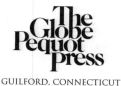

GUILFORD, CONNECTICUT

Text design: Nancy Freeborn

Special thanks to David Emblidge who conceived of this book and helped streamline it to perfection.

Many thanks for the photo contributions of Organic Valley Family of Farms: pages 28, 34, 40, 48, 74; Pete and Gerry's Organic Eggs: pages 44, 67, 70; Transfair/Magnum Photos: page 12; and Evergreen Wheatgrass: page 5.

Library of Congress Cataloging-in-Publication Data
Meyerowitz, Steve.
    The Organic Food Guide / Steve Meyerowitz.
        p. cm.
    Includes bibliographical references and index.
    ISBN 0-7627-3069-2
        1. Natural foods. 2. Organic gardening. I. Title.

TX369.M48 2004
641.5'63—dc22   2004040617

Manufactured in the United States of America
First Edition/First Printing

contents

What nature delivers to us is never stale.

Because what nature creates has eternity in it.

–Isaac Bashevis Singer (1904–1991)

INTRODUCTION

Food. It's the one thing we all have in common. We eat. And we do it every day, many times per day. There are so many decisions—what to eat, where to eat, when to eat, with whom to eat—and it's getting worse. Now we have to decide what to buy and where to shop. It used to be a simple case of apples vs. oranges. Nowadays it's getting hard to compare apples to apples!

A casual walk down the grocery aisle proves it. These days you could get lost in there! There are so many signs, so many new and different labels, you might as well be walking through Times Square with neon lights flashing at you from every direction! It's not just that there are a lot of products. It's worse; there are a lot of new types of products.

Call it the invasion of the health nuts. It used to be that butter was bad and margarine was good. Today butter has been vindicated, but margarine remains at large. Eggs used to be just white or brown. Now, they are fertile vs. infertile, free-range vs. indoors, natural vs. organic . . . . Apples were always a little confusing—Granny Smiths, McIntoshes, Golden Delicious, Idareds. But now they're also pesticide-free, all natural, locally grown, USDA Organic, California Organic, International Certified, and Biodynamic, not to mention the familiar "conventional." It's a tangled jungle of jumble out there! They say an apple a day keeps the doctor away, but shopping for one can give you a headache!

Sure, it's a little confusing—all the different varieties of apples and their alternatives. But variety is healthy, just like competition is healthy. Competition is also good for prices. With organic foods, you'll see good prices and some high prices. But as you will learn in the "Price" chapter, price isn't everything. Quality counts for something, too! And the good news is that with the crazy ups and downs of modern-day marketing, quality does not automatically cost more. Even when it does, many people think it's worth it for food that tastes better. The "Taste" chapter reveals the results of our taste test.

Our food is supposed to be healthy, safe, and nutritious, right? Of course. And it is . . . in the main. But government regulators are not exactly guardian angels. Becoming a truly savvy shopper means educating yourself and your family on issues of concern, and there are some big ones involving health and nutrition. Stay tuned for the two chapters about the health and nutrition values of organic foods.

How did we get here? The development of modern chemical-based agriculture, with its powerful corporate influences and poorly enforced government regulations, is an incredible story. How did these chemicals get into our soil, our food, our bodies, in spite of the hazards? How did the organic movement get to be as big as it is? You can read about its origins in the third chapter.

Admittedly, the result of all these changes to our food supply is making shopping more complex. Maybe you've got ten minutes to pick up three items. But now those three items each have two to three alternatives to choose from. Great. Now you need to add a fourth item—aspirin! What are the real differences between organic and conventional foods besides price? How do "all natural" and "locally grown" compare? What's the difference between fair-trade coffee and regular coffee? We all need to be educated about these issues, which are discussed in the first chapter.

But even if you already know what it means when an apple is labeled organic or Biodynamic, you still have to find it. Sometimes organic and nonorganic foods are shelved side by side, and sometimes the organics are located separately in another part of the store. Sure, there are signs, but how do you identify these foods when you're traveling from store to store? What do the labels look like—the ones for "organic food," "all natural food," "locally grown food"? What do they say? What do they mean? Where are they located on a cereal box, on a bottle of milk, a piece of fruit? You can find all these answers in the "Reading the Labels" chapter, the heart of this book.

This shopping trip may have started out confusing, but on the other side of the coin, it can also be quite interesting. Learning about new types of foods is exciting and fun. Think of it as your first visit to a new neighborhood. Granted, it's a little scary at first, and getting lost there would be a headache. But what if you had your own personal tour guide? Then the frazzle and frustration could be replaced with the joys of a journey where you meet new foods and friends, learn new things, and feel good about doing something positive for your health.

Well, your tour guide has arrived. Rev up your shopping cart. We're headed for a delicious adventure.

What's Organic?

SOME OTHER NATURAL ALTERNATIVES

*He who does not mind his belly, will
hardly mind anything else.*
–Samuel Johnson (1709–1784)

When you walk into a food market these days, it can be like landing at a foreign airport. Which way do you turn? Decisions must be made. It's more than a matter of just locating the items on your list. Nowadays you must decide what *type* of food to buy. Should you get the standard "conventional" food or try the "organic" food? Or should you consider some of the other "natural" alternatives?

You probably already know about conventional food because it's the type most commonly found in the supermarket. (We will explore it further in Chapters 3 and 4.) For now, let us look at just what "organic" is. The terms *organic* and *natural* do not mean the same thing, so we will compare these two types of foods to each other and to conventional food. Once we're clear on what "organic" is, we'll go on to investigate some of the other "natural" alternatives, which include locally grown foods, Community Supported Agriculture (CSA), Biodynamic farming, integrated pest management (IPM), and fair trade.

WHAT IS ORGANIC FOOD?

You could say that the simple definition of *organic,* both the food and the farming system, is that it's antichemical. It's true that organic farmers must keep their plants, soil, and water free of chemicals. But in order for them to put the organic label on their vegetables, quite a number of other conditions must be met. We will explain the requirements and interpretation of the organic insignia in the next chapter. But you can bet that organic farmers do a lot more than just omitting pesticides.

The life of an organic farmer is filled with detailed record keeping, testing and retesting, and surprise inspections. Organic farmers must meet strict standards and reveal their books whenever inspectors inquire. The land must also be free of chemical residues for a minimum of three years. No sewage sludge for fertilizer, no growth hormones or antibiotics are allowed. It's no easy game, especially in these times when genetically modified organisms and pesticide sprays may be flying downwind. Even after organic food leaves the farm, the records must demonstrate that it was transported without ever mingling with non-organic food and that the packaging was not tainted, treated, or irradiated. It's not easy.

Definition of Organic

Organic food is grown, processed, and packaged without the use of agricultural chemicals, artificial colors or flavors, genetic modification, irradiation, or other synthetic ingredients.

Organic farming treats plants, soil, and animals with natural products instead of synthetic chemicals and drugs.

But there's more. Organic food and organic farming represent a philosophy that goes beyond just the quality of food. It strives to maintain the integrity of the entire food chain—plants, soil, air, water, animals, and people. We are all part of the same ecosystem. Food does not come from supermarkets. It is only displayed there. Food comes from the land and from the animals living on the land. Fertile land grows healthier plants for healthier animals and healthier people. Organic farmers aspire to manage all these elements harmoniously. They are convinced that nutritious vegetation can be produced only by putting back into the soil what was taken out and that "green" (ecologically sound) manures and compost do a better job of that than synthetic fertilizers. In their view, crops grown under organic methods are sufficiently pest- and disease-resistant without the use of chemicals, and the risks of chemicals in agriculture far outweigh the advantages.

Organic farmers believe that although pesticides produce abundant amounts of low-cost food, they create higher costs in other sectors of society. The food is cheap, but the cleanup is exorbitant. Consumers may save at the supermarket, but they lose these savings through tax dollars, agribusiness sub-sidies, and superfunds—all necessary to correct the results of chemical-based agriculture. The time, expense, and trouble devoted to restoring clean air, water, and soil—in this generation and the next—is greater than any advantages pesti-cides provide. Not only that, organic farmers argue that because rising demand from consumers is driving prices downward, organic products can better com-pete against conventional production.

At heart, organic farmers are stewards of the land and managers of sustainable agriculture. This means they want the land to be viable for growing food for future generations. The small family farm, once the foundation of American society, is threatened with extinction. Whole industries such as steel, textile, and mining have disappeared from North America. They have become imports. Will wholesome food become another imported product? Organic farmers, and all promoters of sustainable agriculture, want to prevent our children from inheriting a planet in cri-sis with toxic waste and global warming. Instead they want to create a legacy of fertile land that will produce healthy food for future generations.

Organic Treatment of the Soil

One of the basic principles of organic farming is to recycle and replenish the resources used. Nowhere is this idea more apparent than in how the soil is fertilized. Synthetic fertilizers are con-centrated salts and minerals that can result in an overabundance of nitrogen and phosphorous in the ground. They are petroleum industry by-products that may even contain industrial waste. The organic gar-dener, instead, enriches the soil with cover cropping and composting.

organic Gardening Techniques

Cover cropping is the plant-ing of legumes and grasses on the land for a season instead of vegetables. Cover crops enrich the soil by depositing their nitrogen and allowing the land to recoup its nutrients.

Composting is the recycling of organic matter back into soil. The building blocks of compost are lawn clippings, garden waste, shredded newspaper, vegetable scraps (but no meat scraps), manure, leaves—most anything from your garden and kitchen. These materials decay with the assistance of air, water, earthworms, and bacteria into a dark, nutrient-rich mixture that will enrich and replenish exhausted soil.

Organic Treatment of Insects and Pests

Balance and prevention are central to the philosophy of organic farming. All elements in the garden should work in balance with one another, and that includes insects. But the domination of insects over plants is not accepted. Thus, if some beetles are munching on the potato leaves, the organic farmer is willing to allow a small donation of that crop to the beetles. But a conventional farmer plants acres upon acres of potatoes, invariably creating an out-of-control beetle population that can be managed only by extraordinary measures—chemicals. The organic farmer, instead, alternates potato fields with other vegetable crops so the hungry beetle never dominates. That's prevention.

Organic farmers use their tools and tricks to outsmart the bugs. They place netting and row covers on the crops to block insect entrance. They use 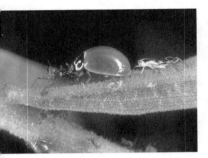 sticky pheromone traps to lure insects with the scent of the opposite sex. They repel insects with sprays made from soaps, oils, hot pepper sauce, and garlic. Natural bacterial solutions, such as *Bacillus thuringiensis,* stop caterpillars, especially on kale, cabbage, broccoli, and other brassicas. It is nontoxic to everything else and is readily available at most garden centers.

Natural predators are the organic farmer's best friends. Birds, bats, frogs, lizards, spiders, and ladybugs are invited into the garden to eat the bugs. Tiny parasitic wasps protect the garden by eating small worms and insect eggs. Small blossoming plants such as sweet alyssum and dill attract beneficial insects with their sweet nectar. Pesticides, on the other hand, kill these beneficial predators as well as the insects.

Organic Treatment of Fungus and Disease

Plants, like people, are exposed to elements in the environment that might make them sick. The most common are fungal infections. Fungicides are the botanical equivalent of antibiotics. They fight plant disease. The conventional farmer sprays fungicides to prevent disease. The organic farmer, on the other hand, shelters plants from the conditions that promote disease and selects disease-resistant varieties.

Like a hawk, an organic farmer develops a keen sense of observation. Organic farmers know that high moisture and low air circulation promote fungus growth. So, they plant with adequate room for growth between plants instead of packing them tightly to conserve acreage. The more room there is, the more air circulation and sun, and thus lower moisture buildup and mold.

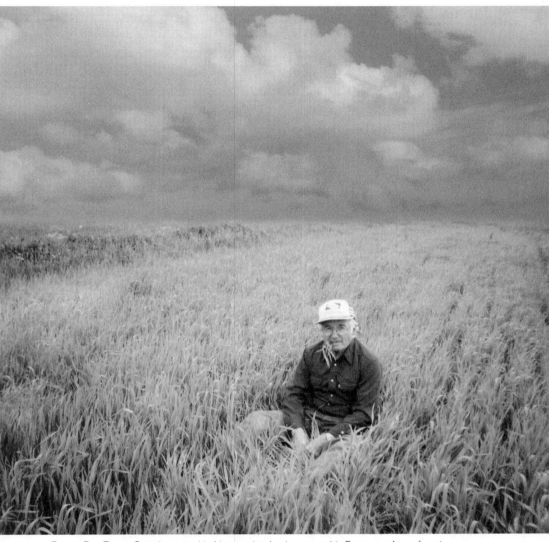

Farmer Dan Tomen Sr. enjoys a rest in his organic wheat grass on his Evergreen Acres farm in Wardsville, Ontario, Canada. COURTESY EVERGREEN WHEATGRASS

Seed selection is also key. Organic farmers choose hardy varieties that survive in difficult conditions. Picking plants that adapt better to the local climate and conditions means they don't need a lot of attention. This adaptation is analogous to people who have stronger immunity to certain diseases. Again, this is the principle of prevention. If a plant does catch a disease, the farmer removes it immediately so it cannot spread.

Organic Treatment of Weeds

Weeds challenge farmers every day, providing one of the most labor-intensive aspects of farming. That is why herbicides, or "weed killers," are so popular. Organic farmers have been spraying weeds with cider vinegar for years. Now scientists at the U.S. Agricultural Research Service have made it official. Vinegar successfully kills weeds such as lamb's-quarters, giant foxtail, velvetleaf, smooth pigweed, and the notoriously stubborn Canada thistle.

Organic farming is a little like baseball. Organic farmers never know what kind of pitch nature is going to throw. They have to be ready for anything. That's why they continually educate themselves and keep up with the latest techniques. Organic farmers don't believe in conquering nature; rather, they strive to coexist with it. Their philosophy is simple: Plant more than you need. The insects eat some, and we eat the rest.

Key Points about Organic Food

- Healthier and more nutritious
- No pesticide risks
- Safer for children
- Cleaner air, water, and soil
- Locally grown food is fresher and tastier
- Protects the environment
- Preserves long-term use of land

SOME OTHER NATURAL ALTERNATIVES

What Does "Naturally Grown" Mean?

Here's a riddle. It's not organic, but it's natural. Can you figure this one out? Organic is all naturally grown, right? Yes! But all naturally grown is *not* necessarily organic.

Confusing? Yes, because there are no regulations, and therefore there is no universal definition of the term "naturally grown." Organic farmers have rules covering what they are permitted to do in order to control pests, improve the soil, manage the weeds, feed the animals, and so forth. The *Manual of Organic Standards* is many pages long, and there is a penalty if you violate it. Surprise visitors show up from time to time. They're called inspectors! They walk the farm, feel the soil, test the water, look in the Dumpster, and sniff the compost. After that, they kick the mud off their shoes and snoop around the office looking at receipts for feed, seed, fertilizer, traps, lures, repellents, and other records, reports, and tests. All of this paperwork gets logged, sorted, and reported. If all your Ts are crossed, you get a certificate authorizing use of the organic label. That's where the money part comes in. To do this twice per year takes time and costs money. Somebody has got to pay, and it's the organic farmer. Ouch!

This record keeping is a necessity for farms wanting to market with the organic insignia. But it is so expensive and time consuming that only the larger farms with a national market can afford it. It is too expensive and unmanageable for smaller farmers like the ones you meet at the local farm stands and markets. Unlike national farms that specialize in a few crops and sell to chain stores and processing plants, small farmers typically grow a little bit of everything, from vegetables to fruits to flowers. Their outlets are farmers' markets, local restaurants, and grocers.

Enforcement is necessary. The U.S. National Organic Program (NOP) requires all producers who sell more than $5,000 of goods per year—in other words, bigger than a backyard operation—to be certified. Violators can be fined as much as $10,000 per incident. This protection is necessary to stop cheaters and prevent corruption.

organic vs. Natural

Organic food is packaged and processed without the use of additives or preservatives and grown without pesticides or genetic modification. From farm to table, the process is monitored and certified.

Natural food is packaged and processed without the use of additives or preservatives, but it may be grown using some conventional methods, including pesticides and genetically engineered grain. There is no authorized monitoring or certification.

Naturally Grown—Ideal for Small Farmers

What are small farmers to do if they can't afford to join the NOP? The only thing they can do is to describe their products as "naturally grown." Unfortunately, "naturally grown" is unregulated. You never know exactly what you are getting when you see the sign NATURALLY GROWN. Can we assume it means "without pesticides"? Was the soil nourished with compost? Did the chickens roam free? There is no guarantee. Many small farmers who identify their products this way do practice sustainable farming, use fewer pesticides, and even employ some organic methods. Nevertheless, even if they follow 100 percent of the organic rules, they would need to go through the certification process in order to use the word "organic." The good news is that because they are small, you may have the opportunity to meet and talk to them. They will tell you directly how they farm, and you can decide whether or not to believe them!

Many small farmers are still committed to following the organic rules even if they cannot afford to do so officially. The problem for us consumers is that there are no guarantees. That is the downside of no regulation. Some small farmers are trying to do something about this by certifying one another. A group called Certified Naturally Grown are essentially organic farmers in disguise. They have created their own no-cost, nonprofit, certification program wherein farmers inspect other farmers once per year. They follow the national organic rules and post their inspection reports on the Internet. Although not federally approved, these farmers are a step above other "natural" farmers because the program adds credibility to their efforts. You can even view a list of the approved (and rejected) farms. To learn more, visit the Web site www.naturallygrown.org.

Comparison: Conventional, Natural, and Organic

Processing	Conventional	Natural	Organic
Artificial Flavors	Allowed	No	No
Artificial Colors	Allowed	No	No
Artificial Preservatives	Allowed	No	No
Farming			
Certification	No	No	Yes
Artificial Fertilizers	Allowed	Allowed	No
Synthetic Pesticides	Allowed	Allowed	No
Irradiation	Allowed	Allowed	No
Gene Modification	Allowed	Allowed	No

Locally Grown

No matter how "natural" it is or isn't, naturally grown produce is often locally grown. Locally grown produce has certain advantages: It is in season, there is no trucking or refrigeration, its low distribution costs make it economical, and it is usually fresher. That freshness often translates into great taste. And it's nice to know your purchases are supporting your local economy.

When Grandpa was alive, 85 percent of his diet came from near his home. Today the situation has totally flipped: 85 percent of our diet is shipped in from distant growers and often from 3,000 miles away. Sure, some transportation of food is necessary, but we have become overly dependent on this global delivery network. Agricultural policies today favor factory farms, giant supermarkets, and long-distance trade. But if we were to spend our money on locally grown foods, those dollars would likely stay in the region, create jobs, and buy local goods and services. Small organic and local farms help the environment and preserve the character and beauty of a community.

Key Points about Locally Grown Food

- Food is often fresher, tastier, and in season
- Connects us to our food chain
- Supports family farms
- Preserves open spaces
- Helps local economy
- Builds community

Even chain store supermarkets are starting to understand the benefits of locally grown foods. They appreciate that food comes directly from the producer to their market. And they understand the public relations value of telling their customers about how they are helping preserve the family farm in a region that loves its local farm history. They can proclaim to their customers that they are preserving those beautiful rolling hills and lush green valleys. They also recognize the economic advantage for all concerned—farmer, supermarket, and consumer. Local farmers, however, do not enjoy the advantages of economy of scale to sell their products to the distributors at profitable margins. But by going directly to supermarkets, they eliminate intermediaries, and even the supermarkets benefit by a lower price. The consumer gains by getting a fresher product at a better price. Eliminating all those shipping and handling bills for cross-country food transportation saves a bundle. It's a win-win situation.

CSA—Community Supported Agriculture

As its name implies, Community Supported Agriculture is a marriage between consumer and farmer. Unlike most farms, this one is "not-for-profit." Each CSA has a circle of subscribers who agree in advance to meet the financial needs of the farm. In return they receive a "share" of the harvest as the season arrives.

This arrangement guarantees the farm and farmer enough financial support to keep these small and medium-size farms in business. In addition, it keeps farms in the community and maintains local food sources. These farms are typically organic, but they may also be in transition to organic or use low-chemical input. In any case, the food won't include a premium to pay for third-party certification. This is one case where the consumer knows everything about how the food was produced. Members even volunteer (optional) to help out on the farm. No insignia necessary here. You know exactly what you are getting.

A "share" typically costs a family between $300 and $600 and serves a family for a full season or a full year. Members usually visit once per week to pick up their more-than-ample allotment. Some CSAs also incorporate a food buying club through which members use their collective buying power to obtain nonlocal foods and dry goods. Through good seasons and bad, CSA members remain faithful to their farms. Farmers don't have to worry about anything except farming, and members benefit from the experience of living closer to their food and to the earth.

The concept of community supported farming was first developed in Switzerland and Japan. The first CSA in North America was Indian Line Farm of South Egremont, Massachusetts, started in 1984 by Robyn Van En. Today there are more than 1,000 CSAs in the United States alone. To find a CSA farm near you, visit the CSA Web site, www.CSAcenter.org.

Key Points about CSAs

- Not-for-profit private farm serving its members
- Typically organic, but not always
- Fresh, nutritious, affordable, wholesome
- Good for local economy
- Supports sustainable agriculture
- Direct link from farm to table
- No costly long-distance food dependency

Biodynamic Farming

Biodynamic farming is organic farming with a cosmic connection. The Biodynamic gardener is a farmer who aspires to integrate organic methods with the rhythms of the sun, moon, planets, and stars. A Biodynamic farm is a self-contained unit where the animals maintain the fertility of the farm and the farm in turn maintains the animals. On a Biodynamic farm, the animals, farmers, and families live according to the examples of self-sufficiency that nature provides.

Biodynamics is part of the work of Rudolf Steiner, an early-twentieth-century teacher who described the earth as a living being and proposed that agriculture was more than just an assemblage of techniques. In his philosophy, farming was an ongoing path of higher knowledge in which the farmer learns to read the language of nature—the "science of life forces"—which includes everything that affects plant growth. Biodynamics results in health and balance for all who live on the farm—people, plants, and animals—by achieving harmony with nature.

Key Points about Biodynamic Farming

- Certified organic food with a cosmic connection
- Planting, cultivating, and harvesting is done according to the natural rhythms of the sun, moon, planets, and stars
- Soil health is intimately connected to plant life
- Self-sufficient farming environment
- Sustainable agriculture with recycling and composting
- Principles and philosophy take priority, not profit
- Based on the philosophy of Rudolf Steiner

IPM—Integrated Pest Management

Integrated Pest Management describes a program of reduced pesticide use based on pest identification and monitoring and ecological controls. In short, it is a more controlled and conservative approach to pesticide use than that of conventional farms. A key tenet of IPM is the selection of pesticides with the lowest risk to the public and the environment. IPM farms can use 30 to 50 percent fewer pesticides than conventional farms.

Several states have IPM programs, which serve as an information and education service for farmers. They are closely aligned with the agricultural departments of major universities. There is no nationally coordinated IPM program or labeling.

Key Points about IPM

- Not organic
- Lower pesticide residues
- Increases availability of safer, local produce
- Regional standards established by states and agricultural universities
- Incorporates some sustainable, ecological methods

IPM is an admirable effort to reduce pesticide use. How do they do it? By incorporating some methods used by organic farmers. IPM growers use crop rotation and cover crops, disease-resistant seeds, and natural controls such as beneficial insects and pest barriers. But it is a far cry from organic. There is no national program for verification or labeling. There are no standards for prohibited or allowed pesticides. And, as of this writing, there is no position on genetically engineered foods. But IPM does recognize the potential risks of pesticide usage on the environment and public health and offers education and training to conventional farmers who wish to reduce pesticide use. National IPM labeling may eventually be established. To get the latest news about this program, contact the IPM Institute of North America at www.ipminstitute.org.

Fair Trade

Much of the food network involves international trade. Foods like bananas, pineapples, coffee, and chocolate often come from poor, tropical, developing nations far away from the industrial world. More and more foods, such as sugar, honey, oranges, and even flowers are coming from these countries because of their extremely low-cost labor. Unfortunately, while residents of the United States may be enjoying a $4 latte at Starbucks, some of the Latin American growers responsible for those beans cannot afford to send their children to

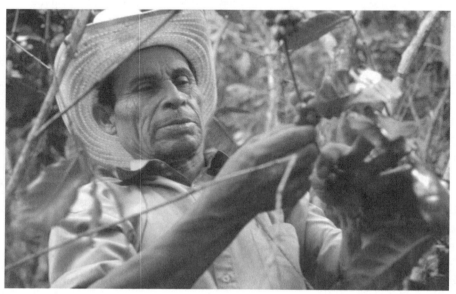

Santiago Rivera, a member of the Fair Trade cooperative "Prodecoop," picks ripe coffee cherries on his farm in the Segovias region of Nicaragua. PHOTO © 1999 SUSAN MEISELAS/MAGNUM PHOTOS

school. Many of them also suffer injuries from unprotected use of dangerous pesticides. The inequities of such trade spawned a new movement under which the growers receive premium prices and are trained to follow organic and/or ecologically sustainable farming practices. It's called fair trade.

Key Points about Fair Trade

- Develops honest, fair trade relationships with farmers
- Pays a higher than conventional price
- Trains farmers about sustainable agriculture
- Works directly with farmer co-ops
- Certified organic in some instances

It seems crazy. If fair trade is doable, then why isn't it done universally? Fact is, coffee is big business. Along with chocolate and bananas, it is among the most heavily traded commodities in the world. The chain of events that carries the coffee beans from El Salvador to New York involves a cast of intermediaries—processors, creditors, exporters, brokers—all of whom take their share. Latin American farmers call them "coyotes." Their cut is the difference between the farmers having and not having essentials like food and clothing. The Equal Exchange's annual report of 2003 states that the conventional market price for cocoa was $640 per metric ton in 2000. The fair trade price was $1,950 per ton. The 2002 conventional price for coffee was 45 cents per pound. The fair trade price was $1.26. But because the fair traders represent only a tiny fraction of the coffee trade, coffee farmers exported the majority of their harvest to conventional brokers. Imagine if your income underwent such drastic changes! For many farmers trapped in poverty across Latin America, Africa, and Asia, fair trade represents hope for their communities: hope they will not lose their land and that their children will attend school.

> **The extra money our cooperatives receive makes a difference in medicines and nurseries to care for our children.**
>
> —Mateo Rendon, farmer, El Salvador

Not all foods grown by fair trade cooperatives are farmed organically. Fair trade does not mean organic. But the fair trade program is dedicated to sustainable agriculture. This means that fair trade coffee, chocolate, bananas, etc. are "all natural," if not labeled CERTIFIED ORGANIC.

Fair trade has its own certification program similar in procedure to the organic program, but its focus is on sustainability and fair price. Fair Trade Certified tracks the product through independent, nonprofit, certifying organizations. These organizations, FLO International and TransFair U.S., ensure that the products were bought directly from small, democratically controlled farmer co-ops whose members abide by child labor and other labor laws and are paid a guaranteed minimum price.

A Word about Farmers' Markets

As you stroll through a busy farmers' market, the smell of freshly baked bread pulls you to the left, and the perfume of lilies and hyacinths pulls you to the right. Why, you just might swoon off your feet into that pyramid of apples were it not for the steadying sight of a block of raw cheese, fresh milk in glass bottles, and the pastel-colored eggs in a hay-filled box. Market day is here! And along with its truly eclectic array of offerings, the farmers' market has a distinctive, festive atmosphere that recalls an earlier time when the market was the social center of the town. Here you will find familiar faces and make friends with regulars, farmers and shoppers alike. What could be better than that? Only, perhaps, eating these exquisite foods within hours of their picking!

According to the 2002 Worldwatch Institute report, there were more than 3,100 registered farmers' markets in the United States in 2001, up from 300 in 1975. What is the reason for this tremendous growth? Small farmers locked out of the food distribution network found that they could bypass the distributors and supermarkets and go directly to the consumer and make a good profit while providing local, high quality, affordable food.

Many organic farmers sell at farmers' markets. It is a great outlet for them because they can make a profit and keep prices in line with conventional produce. Most of these farmers are too small to use the organic label. Some grow with organic methods; others use reduced amounts of pesticides. No guarantees here. But you can ask the farmer and you'll probably learn a lot.

Whether you come home with certified organic or just naturally grown foods, shopping at farmers' markets is an enriching experience with superb variety and flavor. Start early in the morning to get the best pickings. You can bet there is a farmers' market near you. Visit the Web site www.localharvest.org.

Reading
The Labels:

WHAT DO THEY MEAN?

We are indeed much more than what we eat,
but what we eat can nevertheless help us
to be much more than what we are.

–Adelle Davis, 1970

In the 1970s, organic food went by many names: "organic," "all-natural," "antibiotic-free," "pesticide-free," "free-range," "ecological," "fair-trade," and so on. Trying to figure out what they all meant was enough to make you run for the aspirin bottle! The only thing you knew for sure was that these products were not conventionally farmed. In spite of the fact that both shoppers and store owners believed in these labels, there was no guarantee. In an effort to protect the good efforts of organic farmers and to prevent fraud, several non-profit organizations emerged that established organic standards. The first of these was the California Certified Organic Farmers (CCOF). Soon, other independent certifying agencies were launched, and several U.S. states began running similar verification programs.

Don't put away that aspirin bottle just yet. The new rules were good, but there were too many of them! With the increasing demand and rising market prices for organic products, the need for universal certification—one standard for everyone to follow—became crucial. In 1990 the U.S. Congress passed the Organic Foods Production Act, which mandated that the U.S. Department of Agriculture (USDA) establish national standards for the growing, processing, and marketing of organic products. These standards were finally implemented in October 2002. During the twelve-year delay, other nations also began to establish uniform rules for what can and cannot be called "organic food."

LABELING RULES FOR ORGANIC PRODUCTS

The rules established by the USDA are essentially equivalent to the organic standards set by many other nations. Basically, they address the methods and substances used in producing organic fruits, vegetables, meats, poultry, and dairy products. These rules prohibit such things as synthetic pesticides, insecticides, artificial fertilizers, antibiotics, and hormones. They also exclude the use of genetically modified organisms (GMOs), fertilization with sewage sludge, and ionizing radiation (irradiation) for extending shelf life. The rules include a list of approved substances such as natural pesticides made with ingredients like soap, garlic, or hot pepper sauce, and biological pest controls that use bacterial solutions.

Food handlers and transporters also have a list of both approved and prohibited substances. They are required to stop the commingling of organic with nonorganic commodities and to prevent contact with prohibited substances. The rules also officially validate and require the use of such age-old organic practices as composting, cover cropping, crop rotation, recycling, soil fertility, tillage, and cultivation practices, as well as the use of natural predators. Livestock must be fed organically produced grain and have access to pasture and free range.

USDA Organic Standards

Prohibited
- No synthetic pesticides, herbicides, fungicides
- No antibiotics or growth hormones
- No sewage sludge or artificial fertilizers
- No GMOs (splicing in genes from other species)
- No irradiation (X-rays and gamma rays to kill pathogens)

Required
- Animals have access to the outdoors
- Livestock fed organic feed
- Crop rotation, composting, recycling
- Land free of chemicals for at least three years
- Nontoxic pest management
- Records, plans, and audit trails maintained

ENFORCEMENT OF STANDARDS

All agricultural products sold, labeled, or represented as organic in the United States must comply with the federal organic law passed in 2002. The USDA has accredited several preexisting certifying agencies, giving them the responsibility of inspecting farms, processing facilities, testing soil and water, and checking the records of producers, processors, and handlers. These agencies also investigate complaints of noncompliance. Violations are punishable by fines of $10,000 per incident. Only farmers who sell less than $5,000 per year and retail food stores that sell the products but do not process them are exempt. Food manufacturers and farmers who pass all the tests are entitled to display the USDA organic seal.

WHO ARE THE "CERTIFYING AGENTS"?

These are the folks who actually go down to the farm or the warehouse to inspect the goods. Somebody has to do the inspecting, and the USDA does not use its own staff for this job. Instead it authorizes independent inspection agencies, including state agencies, to do the job. There are about sixty of these, such as California Certified Organic Farmers (CCOF), Oregon Tilth, Organic Crop Improvement Association (OCIA), Northeast Organic Farming Association (NOFA), and others. Many of these agencies were doing this work for years before federal regulation. Before the National Organic Program (NOP) was established in 2002, these agencies all followed similar rules and controls for certification. However, even small differences created complications for producers selling across state lines and especially across borders. Since 2002 these agencies and foreign certifiers have all become accredited by the USDA. Now everybody follows the same rules.

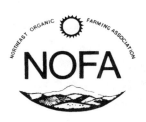 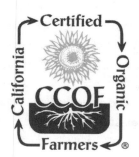 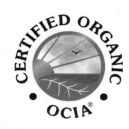

INTERNATIONAL PRODUCTS AND CERTIFICATION

It's a small world. Every grocery store includes products from other countries. France is famous for its wine, Ireland for its beer, Switzerland for its chocolate. In the United States, we even import water! So how is a U.S. program going to label foreign products? Simple. In addition to the U.S.-based certifying agencies, the USDA also authorizes approximately forty foreign certifiers. In other countries, the process is reversed. We'll review the international players later. But first let's examine the U.S. labels.

HOW THE LABELS APPEAR

Where Is the Organic Symbol?

What's on your grocery list? Pizza, applesauce, peanut butter, yogurt, cookies, vitamins, cereal, salad dressing . . . so many different foods and different types of packages. Here's how to find the "organic" information.

Most products display the symbol, or organic seal, in a prominent place on the package. Organic products require a lot of extra work from farm to market, so the majority of organic producers are proud to proclaim the "proof" of their efforts—the organic insignia. The USDA organic seal is typically found on the front of the package but is not required to be there. The producer may choose to put the label on the back of the package. If you don't see it, that may be because the product does not meet the requirements. It must be at least 95 percent organic to show on the label. Sometimes, on older labels, only the symbol of the USDA-authorized certifier is displayed. That agency's emblem is a perfectly acceptable substitute for the USDA seal. In fact, the law does not require the USDA seal to be shown, but it does mandate the presence of the certifier's seal. Thus, at the very least, you will find the certifying agency's seal and the words CERTIFIED ORGANIC BY followed by the certifying agency name. If you can't find it, look at the end of the ingredients list. To see the U.S. National Organic Program, and to get the latest changes in food labeling procedures, go to the Web site www.ams.usda.gov/nop.

Chances are you can put away that aspirin now, or at least set it down. You won't need a magnifying glass, either. There are four levels of organic rules, and they are pretty simple. They start with the most organic (100 percent) and end with the least organic (less than 70 percent). It's a fabulously logical system.

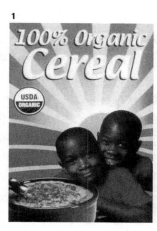

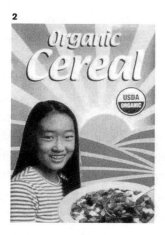

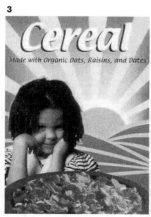

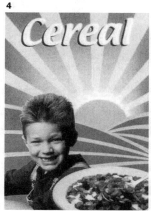

The four categories of the USDA labeling rules. The words on each cereal box describe the percentage of organic ingredients. Boxes 1 and 2, 100 percent and 99–95 percent, include the seal. Boxes 3 and 4, 94–70 percent and less than 70 percent, do not.

Label for Single-Ingredient Foods

Fruits and Vegetables. The USDA organic sticker or the certifier's sticker may appear on unpackaged fruits and vegetables, such as bananas, apples, or broccoli. These foods are obviously 100 percent organic because you can't have one end of a banana organic and the other end not!

Other Single-Ingredient Foods. For foods such as milk, meat, cheese, and eggs, in addition to the USDA or other organic sticker, the carton or package may include the words ORGANIC or CERTIFIED ORGANIC anywhere on the package and identify the USDA-authorized certification agency by name (CERTIFIED ORGANIC BY . . .) and include the agency's seal anywhere on the package.

Label for 100% Organic Packaged Foods

Packaged or prepared foods are multi-ingredient foods. A jar of applesauce, for example, includes more than just apples. The same is true for a box of cereal, a candy bar, a can of soda, even peanut butter—all contain more than one ingredient. If all the ingredients, excluding water and salt, are certified organic, then the product can proudly proclaim 100% ORGANIC prominently on the front of the package. Even in cases where the USDA emblem is not displayed, the words 100% ORGANIC are your assurance that the product is indeed organic. You will also find the words CERTIFIED ORGANIC BY followed by the name of the authorized certifying agency, along with its seal. This seal is mandatory. The USDA made its own seal voluntary. In the majority of cases, however, you will find both seals. Finally, the name and address of the food manufacturer (farmer, distributor, or packer) must be listed here as well. Usually it is on the back after the ingredients list. This format, by the way, is repeated at all four levels of the organic rules.

Label for 95% to 99% Organic

This label is for packaged foods. An apple, for example, can only be 100 percent organic, but applesauce can be 95 to 100 percent organic. As long as 95 percent or more of the ingredients by weight, not including water and salt, are organic, then the product can prominently display the word ORGANIC or the phrase 9X% ORGANIC. You will probably see the USDA organic seal, but it is optional. You will definitely see the emblem of the certifying agency and an ingredients list clearly identifying the organic items, along with the words CERTIFIED ORGANIC BY followed by the certifying agency name and seal. But you will *not* see the claim 100% ORGANIC. Here are some examples. (Note that the following food examples are generic. They do not represent all brands or specific manufacturers. Ingredients in your food purchases may vary.)

Peanut Butter. A jar of one company's organic peanut butter is made with organic peanuts, which represent 98 percent of the product. But the sugar and oil that make up the other 2 percent are not organic. The jar can prominently display the word ORGANIC, since the primary ingredient, organic peanuts, makes up more than 95 percent of its contents. You should also find the USDA organic seal (optional), the emblem of the certifying agency, and the words 98% ORGANIC.

Yogurt. Organic milk is 99 percent of this product, but the enzyme cultures the producer used to make it yogurt are not certified organic. The label therefore can use only the words ORGANIC or 99% ORGANIC, and it must include the certifying agency name and seal. It may also display the USDA seal.

Flavored Applesauce. One brand of cinnamon-flavored applesauce is made with 100 percent certified organic apples, but the cinnamon is not organic. Therefore, the product can use the words ORGANIC or 99% ORGANIC on the jar and must include the certifying agency name and seal. It may also display the USDA seal.

Label for 70% to 94% Organic

Products made with less than 95 percent but more than 70 percent organic ingredients may include the words MADE WITH ORGANIC INGREDIENTS and list the main organic ingredient names on the main display of the package. The percentage of organic content (X% ORGANIC) and the USDA-authorized certifying agent seal may be used on the principal display panel of any product that contains at least 70 percent organic ingredients. If it's not there, look at the end of the ingredients list. The USDA seal, however, is *not* permitted anywhere on the package.

Flavored Yogurt. One brand of strawberry-flavored yogurt is made with organic milk, but the strawberries are not certified organic. Since the strawberries represent 25 percent of this product by weight, the product is only 75 percent organic. Therefore, with less than 95 percent of this product being organic, only the words MADE WITH ORGANIC YOGURT and the certifying agency seal can appear on the label. The USDA organic seal is not permitted on this product.

Pizza. One brand of frozen pizza prominently proclaims MADE WITH ORGANIC STONE GROUND WHEAT. But none of the pizza's vegetable toppings were organically grown. Therefore, this product is less than 95 percent organic by weight. The MADE WITH ORGANIC claim is allowed, but no USDA organic seal is permitted. This product includes another claim, NO GMOs, referring to the omission of genetically modified organisms in the vegetables used. This is good news, but it does not make the vegetable toppings organic, since it represents only one of the requirements for organic certification.

Cookies. The cookies manufactured by a given company are made with organic whole wheat flour, but none of the other ingredients—butter, sugar, molasses, ginger—is organic. Therefore, the product is less than 95 percent organic. The use of the words MADE WITH ORGANIC WHOLE WHEAT FLOUR may be prominently displayed on the package, but not the USDA organic seal. Look for the certifying agency name and insignia instead.

Supplements. This particular dietary supplement contains only one ingredient—organically grown freeze-dried wheatgrass juice powder. This is a whole-food nutritional supplement, which means that only wheatgrass (a food) is encapsulated in the vegetarian capsules. However, since the grass powder is so light, the capsule represents 20 percent of the product weight. Gelatin capsules, made from animal bones and tissues, are approved by the NOP, but (as of the time of this writing) vegetarian capsules are not. Therefore, even though the content of the capsule is 100 percent certified organic, the product may only claim MADE WITH ORGANIC WHEATGRASS. It may not show the USDA seal. The same manufacturer also makes a bottle of bulk grass powder, which is made with the same ingredient found in the capsules. That product can use the words 100% ORGANIC and can show the USDA organic seal.

Label for Less than 70% Organic

We're almost done. This last category is for products that have some organic ingredients, but the total organic content is less than 70 percent of the product, not including water or salt. Don't expect to find the word ORGANIC in big letters on this package. Prominent use of the word ORGANIC is forbidden. You won't find any organic emblems from anybody on this package, either. Certifying insignias are prohibited. But you may find the words X% ORGANIC INGREDIENTS, and the specific organic ingredients will be identified in the ingredients list. Here are some examples.

Mustard. A jar of yellow mustard is made with organic mustard seed, but there is no word ORGANIC on the front label. Why? The mustard ingredients listed are: "water, vinegar, organic mustard seed, salt, spices." Even though this mustard is made with organic mustard seed, it turns out to be less than 70 percent of the product weight. Therefore, the word ORGANIC cannot be used on the front label nor can any organic insignia be displayed. However, use of the word "organic" is permitted in the ingredients listing to identify the mustard seed as an organically grown ingredient.

Salad Dressing. This particular balsamic vinaigrette salad dressing claims ALL NATURAL INGREDIENTS, and the ingredients list includes "organic olive oil." But the other ingredients are not organic. Since the olive oil makes up less than 70 percent of this product, the word ORGANIC can be used only in the ingredients listing. There are no organic insignias to be found.

Cereal. This manufacturer's cereal is made with organic oats. They are the very first ingredient on the list, indicating that the oats are the dominant ingredient in the recipe. However, there is no statement proclaiming MADE WITH ORGANIC OATS. That is allowed only if the product volume is greater than 70 percent organic. In this case, none of the other ingredients listed is organically grown: "wheat flakes, millet flakes, dried raisins, whole wheat flour, rye, barley, dates, wheat germ, hazelnuts, dried apples, bananas, almonds." It turns out that the organic oats content represents only 40 percent of this cereal. The food producers are permitted to say 40% ORGANIC because the organic oats are the dominant ingredient. Nonetheless, since less than 70 percent of the total product is organic, the word ORGANIC can be used only to identify the organic items in the ingredients list. There are no insignias, and there is no prominent use of the word ORGANIC.

Other Label Claims and Their Definitions

Well, you're . . . almost done. You have completed your course in the four major categories of the organic rule with honors. But you have not graduated, not yet! Actually, that was the easy part. Because organics are regulated, the definitions are clear, and there are distinct boundaries separating the different degrees of "organicness." But what about all the other health claims we see these days on the supermarket shelves? Few of them are federally regulated, and their definitions can stump even the likes of Sherlock Holmes.

All Natural. This is a perfect example of an unregulated description. It implies no preservatives, artificial flavors, colors, or other synthetic additives. In other words, applesauce made with just apples, cinnamon, and sugar may be described as "all natural" because there are no preservatives or artificial flavors. But this claim does not provide any information about how the apples were cultivated. Even apples sprayed with pesticides can be identified as "natural" because they are not manufactured or synthetic. Apples are not like Jell-O or cupcakes, which are manufactured in kitchens or bakeries. Apples are made by nature, or at least by trees, so they are "all natural."

100% Natural Ingredients. This is another unregulated claim with the same implications as "all natural." It does *not* imply any organically grown ingredients.

Wild. Fish, seaweeds, and herbs are sometimes described as "wild," because they are not cultivated. That is, no farming methods, either organic or conventional, are used. These products are just grown "in the wild." Thus, no agricultural chemicals were used, but there is no verification, either, so these foods are not "organic." "Wild" is an "all-natural" state.

Certified Naturally Grown. This is an independent effort by a volunteer, nonprofit organization to identify small, local farmers who follow the organic rules but cannot afford to participate in the national organic certification program described in the first chapter. If you see this label, it means the product, usually fresh produce, is as good as organic. The certifying organization is not affiliated with any federal program. For more information check out the Web site www.naturallygrown.org.

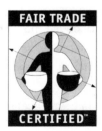

No Preservatives. This is an unregulated claim meaning that common preservatives such as nitrates, nitrites, BHT, sulfites, and the like are not part of the ingredients.

Antibiotic-Free. This is an unapproved and unverified claim. It is also unclear. The USDA actually does sanction two similar claims: "no antibiotics administered" and "raised without antibiotics." The implication is that these meat and poultry producers did not use antibiotics in their animal feed. But even though the USDA is accountable for proper use of these claims, it presently has no verification system in place. Only organic-labeled meats are verified to be antibiotic-free.

rBGH Free. A statement such as "made with rBGH-free cheese" is not a regulated claim. It refers to the use of bovine growth hormones in dairy cows. Certified organic cheese has the only verified rBGH-free claim. Prohibition of hormones, however, is only one element of organic certification. Such a claim, by itself, does not fully meet organic criteria.

Fair Trade Certified. This is an alternative economic and marketing program for farmers in developing countries. It strives to protect the viability of small-scale farmers, maintain sustainable agriculture, and pay fair wages. The top fair trade products are coffee, tea, and chocolate. The fair trade insignia is not an organic label, but it does identify these foods as having achieved certain high standards. For more information visit the Web site www.transfairusa.org.

Free-Range. A partially regulated, general claim implying that a meat or poultry product, including eggs, comes from an animal raised in the open air or that was free to roam. The USDA regulates this claim for poultry only, not beef or eggs.

Biodynamic. A regulated and approved claim that defines a certified organic food that meets additional standards beyond regular organics (see previous discussion in the first chapter). Only one certifying agency, the Demeter Association, inspects Biodynamic foods. Look for the Demeter Biodynamic seal.

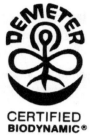

CERTIFIED
BIODYNAMIC®

International Organic Certification

If you've survived the organic foods indoctrination this far, then get out your cap and gown: You deserve a royal graduation—unless you plan to do some shopping or eating outside the United States. In that case, there are a few more things you need to know.

Organic agriculture is currently practiced in more than 120 countries; it's a global business. While the United States hosts the largest organic market in the world (in terms of dollars), the International Federation of Organic Agriculture Movements (IFOAM) says there are many other countries that have greater percentages of devoted organic consumers and more organic acreage. In Austria, Sweden, and Switzerland, organic agriculture accounts for 10 percent of the farmed land. In Germany, 60 percent of shoppers said they buy organic foods occasionally. Italy has more than 60,000 organic farmers, and Australia has more acreage devoted to organic farming than any other country.

In order for products from other countries to be considered verified organic, governments must have a system in place that endorses the certifiers. Just as the USDA accredits independent certifying agencies to verify the growing, processing, and distribution conditions of U.S.-grown products, it has a similar accreditation program in place for imports. Since all countries import and export, most trading programs include verification of organic commodities based on equivalent standards. There are three groups that make international organic trade possible: government agencies, trade associations, and international certifying agents.

Government Agencies

Like the USDA, the government agency for the United States, there are centralized programs in other countries that provide the same service of authorizing domestic certifying agencies. These national organic programs maintain the continuity of standards both within their country and with other countries that is essential for international trade. Here are just a few of the key players.

Australia. Australian Quarantine and Inspection Service (AQIS) is the government authority that accredits the Australian Certified Organic (ACO) agency to carry out certification of products and producers in domestic and international markets. For details see the Web site www.bfa.com.au.

Canada. The Standards Council of Canada authorizes all the certifying agencies in Canada to follow its Canadian Organic Standards (COS). Canada is one of the world's largest suppliers of organic grains and oil seeds such as safflower. For more information see the Web site www.agr.gc.ca.

European Union. The European Union has a dedicated organic consumer population that spends almost as much on organic food as the United States (about 10 billion Euros [US$12 billion] in 2000) and has four times more acreage devoted to organic farming than the United States does. With its fifteen core member nations and a dozen new applicants, the EU could eventually surpass the United States as the leader of the organic movement. Whenever you see the green EU organic seal, you can be certain that at least 95 percent of the product is made with organic ingredients. Further information is available online at europa.eu.int/comm/agriculture/qual/organic.

Japan. The Japanese Agricultural Standard (JAS) for Organic Agricultural Products is the government body that regulates the labeling of organic products for Japan. For details check the Web site www.maff.go.jp.

United Kingdom. The Advisory Committee of Organic Standards (ACOS) is the UK government authority responsible for the approval and supervision of organic certification agencies. The leading certifier in the United Kingdom is the Soil Association Certification Ltd., which certifies 80 percent of the organic food sold in that country. Its Web site is www.soilassociation.org.

Trade Organizations

The International Federation of Organic Agriculture Movements (IFOAM) is a nonprofit, democratically run organization founded in 1972 that can be described as the coordinator of the worldwide organic agriculture movement. Its handbook, *Basic Standards of Organic Agriculture,* has become the model for certifying organic foods and has been translated into twenty languages. IFOAM accredits the major independent certifying agencies in more than sixty countries and represents the organic 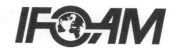 industry at policymaking forums such as the United Nations and the World Trade Organization. It hosts trade fairs and conferences and publishes a magazine, directory, and newsletter. Its directory of 750 organic organizations in 100 countries opens many doors to the world of organic agriculture. The IFOAM Web site is www.ifoam.org.

The Organic Trade Association (OTA) is a membership business association established in 1985 that represents the organic industry in Canada, the United States, and Mexico. It was instrumental in protecting the high standards of the organic industry in the final version of the U.S. National Organic Program. OTA serves as the industry watchdog for governmental agencies and regulators. It also provides a wealth of information to promote organic products and the organic message. The OTA Web site is www.ota.com.

International Certifying Agencies

These are the agencies that go out and do the hands-on work of verification on the farm, in the warehouses, and at the processors, handlers, bottlers, and importers. There are certifiers in more than sixty countries worldwide. One good example is Quality Assurance International. QAI is one of the oldest and largest international certifiers. It is also the leading certifier for U.S. and Canadian products. In addition to certifying farms and manufacturers, QAI also certifies grocers, restaurants, and organic fabrics. Contact IFOAM for a list of certifying agencies by country.

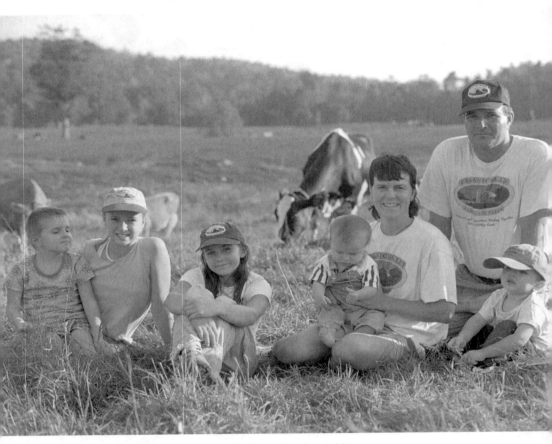

The Varneys make organic farming a family affair on their farm in Maine.

HOW IT ALL BeGan:

ORIGINS OF ORGANIC AGRICULTURE

Your health, happiness, and the future of life on earth
are rarely so much in your own hands
as when you sit down to eat.

—John Robbins, *Diet for a New America*

For generations farmers around the world have been plowing, tilling, and laboring over the land with their sweat and muscle and the savvy that only years of earthy experience brings. Their animals roamed freely, ate healthy grains and grasses, and produced delicious milk and meats.

THE NEW ECONOMICS OF FARMING

Times have changed, however. Although farming was once a highly respected and popular trade, the economics of farming in the modern-day world have forced millions of small family farmers into bankruptcy and converted thousands of acres of pristine farmland into suburban sprawl.

To survive, the remaining farmers had to change. That change came in the 1940s in the form of chemical engineering—modern agricultural products that promised to produce more food on less land, eliminate weeds and insects, and control diseases.

Now there were herbicides to kill weeds, insecticides to kill insects, and fungicides to kill fungus. These chemicals became so popular, they literally transformed farming. The new farming relied less on skill and experience and more on costly chemicals. Small farmers who could not or would not follow the trend eventually went out of business, and the landscape changed. Small towns once adorned with rolling hills and green pastures now grew housing developments, cookie-cutter lawns, and strip malls. If a suburban real estate developer didn't buy the farm, then a multifarm conglomerate did.

According to the USDA, in 1935 there were 6.8 million farms in the United States, but by 2000, only 2.2 million were left. The average size of a farm expanded from 155 acres to 434 acres. These changes—the birth of agribusiness—were driven by the temptations and promises of the new chemical-based agriculture: cheap food and enough to feed the whole world.

TWO INFAMOUS CHEMICALS

DDT—First recognized as a nerve poison for insects in 1939. Used in the fight against malaria. First used as an insecticide in agriculture in 1945. Banned in the United States in 1973. Still in use in some countries today.

Agent Orange—Herbicide (weed killer) famous for its use during the Vietnam War. First developed by Dow Chemical in 1941. Contains 2,4-D (dichlorophenoxyacetic acid), 2,4,5-T (trichlorophenoxyacetic acid), and dioxin. Still in use as a herbicide today.

BIRTH OF THE ORGANIC MOVEMENT

Everybody loves progress, and modern chemical engineering was the high tech of its day. But farmers are, you might say, a firmly grounded breed, and not all of them were convinced that chemistry was good for agriculture. As the marriage of chemistry and agriculture expanded, so too did talk about the dangers of introducing chemicals into our food chain, air, and water. Two British agriculturalists, Sir Albert Howard (*An Agricultural Testament,* 1940) and Lady Eve Balfour (*The Living Soil,* 1943), were the earliest opponents of chemical farm-

> When fertilizers came out in this part of the world in the late 1940s, early 1950s, my dad's first concern was, "Is that going to be good for the land?" He talked to a couple of farmers whose opinions he respected, and he talked to the county agent, and they all assured him that it was. And so he bought the fertilizer attachments, and he bought the fertilizer. He saw his yields go up. And he became a convert like that. I remember him saying, "I could never, ever farm again without fertilizer."
>
> —Farmer Fred Kirschenmann, Jamestown, North Dakota[1]

ing. They developed the concept of composting—that is, using the decaying "organic" matter from grass clippings, leaves, and vegetable scraps to fertilize the soil. This "organic" enrichment of soil became known as "organic farming."

Their writings inspired J. I. Rodale, who published *Organic Farming and Gardening Magazine* (now called *Organic Gardening*) in 1942. Rodale's magazine and his organic research farm, the Rodale Institute in Pennsylvania, did much to popularize "organic" gardening in the United States. By 1954 Helen and Scott Nearing's book, *Living the Good Life,* further inspired the "back-to-the-land" movement that subscribed to eating more fresh, unprocessed foods and growing them with organic gardening methods.

> **For the first time in the history of the world, every human being is now subjected to contact with dangerous chemicals, from the moment of conception until death.**
>
> —Rachel Carson, *Silent Spring,* 1962

But it was biologist Rachel Carson who, in her *Silent Spring* (1962), fired up the organic movement with her shocking exposé of DDT and the harmful effects of pesticides on food, animals, people, and the environment.

The late 1960s was the era of the anti-Vietnam movement, political assassinations, hippies, and increasing cancer rates. Fears about dangerous agricultural chemicals poisoning food and leaching into drinking water were readily added to the zeitgeist by the counterculture—the revolutionary political spirit of the times. The number of organic food supporters grew with every news release of a new pesticide ban.

In 1970 there were two major, organic-related events: The world held its first Earth Day, and U.S. president Richard Nixon established the Environmental Protection Agency. One of the agency's first acts was to ban DDT (1972). It also removed lead from gasoline (1973) and protected drinking water (1974). But it was best known, during the 1970s, for banning several of the most dangerous chemicals the world has ever known: the pesticides Aldrin, Dieldrin, Silvex, and 2,4,5-T. Dioxin was the most lethal ingredient in many of these. The defoliant Agent Orange first made headlines in South Vietnamese newspapers for causing birth deformities. Considered one of the most toxic chemicals of all time, it became emblematic of the public health and environmental dangers of chemical agriculture.

In the 1980s consumers were treated to a smorgasbord of chemical pollution headlines: In Bhopal, India, a leaking insecticide tank killed 2,000 people and injured or permanently maimed 200,000 others. In Love Canal, New York,

237 families had to relocate because chemicals that had been dumped there between 1942 and 1953 were seeping into their homes. In Times Beach, Missouri, so many people and animals were sickened by dioxin contamination that the U.S. government had to purchase all the land and buildings in the town. Added to these headlines were regular news about PCBs, superfund cleanups, endangered species, red dye No. 2, toxic waste, and rising cancer rates.

> **In the United States we've found that everyone's got dioxin in them.**
>
> –Dr. Arnold Schecter, Professor of Preventive Medicine, SUNY Binghamton, 1985

GROWTH OF THE ORGANIC INDUSTRY

In the 1990s organic food and organic farming transformed from a movement into an industry. Organic farming matured beyond the limits of an environmental crusade. Eating safe, untainted food was no longer a radical idea. Rather, it was a rallying point for the masses, one that crossed national borders and economic classes. The bottom line: No one wants to eat poison.

Rising demand in the United States pushed up sales of organic food from $1 billion in 1990 to $5.5 billion in 1998, according to the Organic Trade Association. The industry expanded at a phenomenal 23 percent average annual growth rate. The U.S. Department of Agriculture predicted it would reach $20 billion by 2005. Although North America may have the world's largest appetite for organic food, it is not an American fad. Global sales of organic food were $23 billion in 2002, up 10.1 percent from the previous year. Europe has the world's second-largest organic market, nearly as large as the United States, but areas around the globe are experiencing the tremendous popularity of organic food.

When the USDA recognized and embraced the world of organics in 2002 by adopting a set of uniform standards for labeling organic food, the organic foods industry came of age. This was the first uniform labeling in the world's largest organic market. For consumers its effect was to clarify, expand, and instill in them the confidence that organic foods are what they are purported to be. For the industry its effect was to initiate the mainstreaming of organic foods.

CORPORATE INVOLVEMENT

Organic supporters may have started out as radicals or environmentalists, but they graduated into middle-class, educated shoppers who consider quality when purchasing food. Similarly, organic suppliers may have started out as small entrepreneur-led businesses, but they have grown into medium-size corporations. Meanwhile, the big food industry players are taking notice. They don't want to be left out! As their involvement increases, so does the availability and affordability of organic food. It is this combination of consumer demand and corporate involvement that is making organics accessible to the mainstream in the twenty-first century.

Multinational corporations like McDonald's and Starbucks are going organic. Why? Because it's good for business! McDonald's has an image problem that equates fast food with junk food. In 2002 the company lost money for the first time ever. That's why it started selling organic dairy products (in Europe) and announced in 2003 the phasing out of antibiotic-fed meat products.

> **Demand for organic products is a dynamic consumer trend and Heinz is rising to meet this demand.**
>
> —Justin Lambeth, Heinz

Starbucks, the world's largest coffee corporation, has been targeted by protesters complaining about its use of genetically engineered foods, including milk containing recombinant bovine growth hormone (rBGH). In 2002 it responded by offering organic milk and fair-trade coffee beans in some of its 3,500 stores.

Food giants like Heinz, Dannon, PepsiCo, Pillsbury, Kellogg, General Mills, and Kraft are all going organic by buying up smaller successful organic companies or investing in them. In 2003 Dean Foods, America's largest dairy distributor, bought the largest organic food company in the United States—the dairy collective Horizon Organic. Earlier, M&M-Mars bought the organic food producer Seeds of Change, and General Mills bought organic food companies Cascadian Farms and Muir Glen. The latter acquisition positioned Muir Glen's organic ketchup opposite Heinz. Heinz decided to start its own line of organic ketchup, which was so successful, it added organic spaghetti sauce, baked beans, soups, baby food, and salad dressing. Heinz tells us its expansion into organics was sales-driven. But these mainstream food giants are being caught up in a whirlwind of consumer demand, profits, and good old competition. Thanks in part to the 2002 launch of USDA certification, organic foods are being buoyed on the waves of mainstream capitalism.

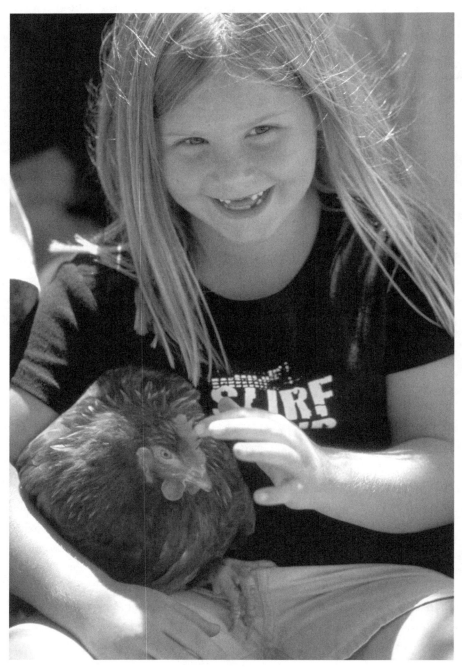

Organic chickens get extra-special attention. COURTESY ORGANIC VALLEY FAMILY OF FARMS

Organic Foods:

HEALTHIER OR NOT?

Health is not valued till sickness comes.
—Dr. Thomas Fuller, 1732

We develop our diets based on a number of considerations: price, cultural tradition, habit, weight loss, taste, convenience, availability, health, and nutrition. More and more people are thinking about health. How do you shop for health? It's not hard. Choosing organics will not eliminate your favorite foods. It merely upgrades the quality of your selections. You still eat the same things, but your shopping priorities now include health, nutrition, and food safety. As a bonus, you get more flavor and that warm and fuzzy feeling that you're doing something good for you, your family, and the planet. More and more people are shopping with health in mind, and organic products are viewed as significant contributors to overall health.

Top Five Motivators for Organic Food and Beverage Purchases

Health and nutrition 66%

Taste 38%

Food safety 30%

Environment 26%

Availability 16%

—Organic Lifestyle Shopper Study 2000, Hartman Group

THE NEW AGRICULTURE

Your great-grandparents ate organic food—although they didn't call it that back then. Before the 1940s there were no pesticides to worry about. Food was just food. Farmers used a lot of manure, and consumers had a lot easier time shopping than we do. Today we don't think about all these pesticides being used to grow our food, nor do we want to. But the reality is they are there and they do influence the purity of our food, air, water, and soil.

Farming has changed. Conventional or modern mainstream farming now includes a big boost from chemical engineering in the form of pesticides, fungicides, insecticides, genetically engineered seeds, and the like. It has changed the culture of agriculture! Farms are bigger, too. Now the average farm is 500 acres. Nobody walks on a farm that size. Only tractor tires touch the soil. It's hard to know what the soil is like without walking on it.

Organic farmers spend a lot of time feeding the soil with things like green manure, humus, and leaves, just like farmers did in the old days. Eventually that soil gets dark and juicy as it becomes rich with nutrients, and those nutrients make their way into our food. The big farms feed the soil, too. But they can't bother with humus and leaves. Agribusiness farmers—the big guys—use synthetic fertilizers spread right from the combine. It's pure nitrate—sodium nitrate, potassium nitrate, and ammonium nitrate. (These chemicals are also used to make nitroglycerin and gunpowder!) It works all right. But the soil is not the same.

It's not common knowledge, but it's no secret either—the majority of these substances are classified as carcinogens. According to the 1997 findings by the Environmental Protection Agency (EPA), the agency that regulates pesticides in the United States, the most popular pesticide groups, the organophosphates and the carbamates, pose the greatest threat to public health. The EPA does not approve or reject these chemicals for human consumption; it only regulates the amount of residues that are permitted to remain on our food.

The EPA's measure of acceptability is at best an imperfect science. After a five-year study in 1993, the National Academy of Sciences condemned the agency's method of establishing tolerances as one based not just on health but also on economic interests. Indeed, many chemicals have been banned, but they were considered safe right up until the day they were removed.

Often it takes a consumer revolt to eliminate these chemicals. Such was the case with Alar on apples. Alar remained on the market for thirteen years after it was identified as a proven carcinogen. Several states banned it, the TV news show *60 Minutes* ran a special report on it, and its manufacturer, Uniroyal, removed it from distribution because of a consumer boycott. All this happened before the EPA finally took action.

Let's face it, we consumers are trusting our government regulators to keep our food safe and healthy. If there are any doubts, the best choice is to go organic.

ORGANIC: THE ALTERNATIVE TO AGROCHEMICALS

Organic food reduces or eliminates the typical health and safety risks associated with modern conventional (chemical) farming. Organically raised cows and chickens don't need antibiotics because they are not packed in tight living quarters—a condition that promotes disease. They roam free. They don't need to be "fattened up" with growth hormones because they are strong and healthy from their diet of green grasses and organic grain. Organic farmers don't need insecticides. They use natural predators such as ladybugs instead or they mix and alternate crops from year to year to prevent the rise of bug populations. Organic farmers build the fertility of the soil with composting and cover cropping to develop nutritious, hardy, disease-resistant fruits and vegetables.

Advantages of Organic Farming

- Produces safer foods
- Produces nutritionally superior foods
- Protects supplies of drinking water
- Keeps rivers, lakes, and streams clean
- Prevents topsoil erosion
- Builds soil fertility
- Protects plant and wildlife habitats
- Uses biodegradable and recyclable materials
- Creates sustainable farmland

HEALTH RISKS OF CONVENTIONAL AGRICULTURE

It's not a savory subject, but it's one you may want to know about. There are health risks in everything we do, even crossing the street. You may not consider eating a "risky business." But the fact is there are proven health hazards in our modern diet, and that is one of the reasons organic food has become so popular. Based on the principle that an informed consumer will be a healthier consumer, the following list briefly describes some of the most controversial health and safety issues created by conventional farming.

Controversial Issues Involving Conventional Food

- Pesticides and public health
- Pesticides in children's diets
- Synthetic fertilizers in drinking water
- Antibiotics and hormones in animal feed
- Factory fish farms
- Genetically modified foods

Pesticides and Public Health

Pesticides have the highest profile of any conventional farming issue. The U.S. Food and Drug Administration (FDA) estimates that twenty pounds of pesticides per person are used every year in the United States. At least fifty-nine of the most popular pesticides are classified as carcinogenic. The prestigious *New England Journal of Medicine* published a study in July 2000 declaring that we are more likely to contract cancer from pesticides and environmental pollutants than from hereditary causes.[1] Medical doctors Landrigan and Needleman in their 1995 book estimated that 80 percent to 90 percent of all cancer in children is caused by exposure to carcinogens in the environment.[2]

It's not good for us, but it's worse for farmers and their families. Because farm workers are exposed to higher levels of these chemicals, their health problems forecast similar troubles for the rest of us. The U.S. National Cancer Institute found that farmers are six times more likely to develop non–Hodgkin's lymphoma than are nonfarmers.[3] Farmers and pesticide application workers also experience higher rates of prostate cancer.[4] According to the U.S. Environmental Protection Agency's own data in 2001, physicians diagnose up to 20,000 pesticide-related illnesses and injuries on farm workers each year.

Thankfully we've banned some of the most dangerous pesticides. But they still linger in our ecosystem. DDT can remain in human tissue for up to fifty years. A Belgian study found that breast cancer patients were five times more likely to show high levels of DDT.[5] Even though DDT was banned from the United States in 1973, it is still in use in less-developed nations. Rural women in Guatemala have shown DDT levels in their breast milk 300 times higher than allowed in the United States.[6]

Pesticides in Children's Diets

If you're a new parent (or can remember when you were one), you probably started cleaning up the family diet in time for the new arrival. With so much controversy about pesticides, that's a good thing. Children are much more susceptible to pesticides because of their low body weights and high metabolisms. In its 1993 report entitled *Pesticides in the Diets of Infants and Children,* the U.S. National Academy of Sciences concluded that government pesticide standards did not protect the health of children. Because of their lesser body weight, up to 35 percent of lifetime exposure to some carcinogenic pesticides occurs by age five.

In a groundbreaking, peer-reviewed study from the University of Washington, children consuming conventional foods showed pesticide residues in their bodies that were six to nine times higher than those who ate organic foods.[7] In 2002 the nonprofit Environmental Working Group called for a ban on the commonly used pesticide methyl parathion. According to the USDA's own data, preschoolers were exceeding government safety limits simply by eating apples and peaches at the same meal.

Researchers at the National Academy of Sciences suggested that one out of four developmental and behavioral problems in children may be linked to pesticides.[8] Protecting children from lead and mercury contamination were hot issues in the 1960s. Perhaps now the time has come to finally protect kids from pesticides.

> **Choosing organic is an easy way to protect our children's health. I buy organic for my children, just like I use seatbelts in our car.**
>
> –Erin Brockovich, environmental activist

Synthetic Fertilizers in Drinking Water

Agrochemicals invade the soil and run into our groundwater. In a 2001 report, the U.S. Geological Survey detected one or more pesticides in more than 90 percent of water and fish samples from streams and in 50 percent of all wells.[9] Nitrates from synthetic fertilizers are another big problem. They form carcinogenic nitrosamines that enter the water table. The big U.S. farm state of Iowa has excessive nitrate levels (greater than 5 ppm) in 30 to 40 percent of its municipal water supplies, according to a University of Iowa study published in 2001. The big risk with nitrates is bladder cancer. Iowa women who drink tap water are nearly three times more likely to develop bladder cancer than those who drink bottled water.[10]

Antibiotics and Hormones in Animal Feed

In case you haven't noticed, very few recipes call for antibiotics. But that's what you're getting when you prepare dishes from beef, chicken, milk, and eggs. According to the Animal Health Institute, an average of 22 million pounds of antibiotics are used annually on livestock. That's twice the amount used by people!

Why so much? It's not all for infections. Conventional livestock farmers serve feed spiked with large amounts of antibiotics and hormones to speed

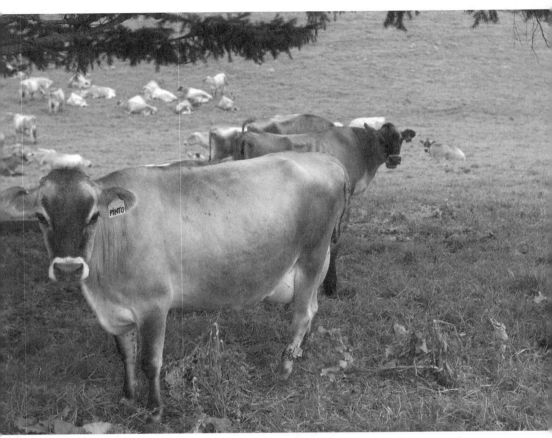

No unhappy cows here at the Bansen farm in Oregon! No antibiotics either. Organic cows roam free, enjoy the open range, and graze on organic grasses. COURTESY ORGANIC VALLEY FAMILY OF FARMS

growth and fatten up their cattle. The result: People are absorbing low-level doses of antibiotics, enabling bacteria to develop resistance to them.

In 1998 the World Health Organization (WHO) recommended an end to the use of human antibiotics in livestock for the promotion of animal growth because of increasing antibiotic-resistant infections in people. Even some of our best drugs, penicillin and tetracycline, are affected, and several strains of pathogenic bacteria with resistance to nearly all known antibiotics have emerged. The problem is so serious that even McDonald's, the world's largest purchaser of beef, announced in 2003 that it was directing its meat suppliers to stop using antibiotic growth promoters.

Factory Fish Farms

Did you know that 90 percent of the salmon sold today is cultivated in fish farms?[11] The days of salmon, shrimp, and tuna caught in the ocean are diminishing due to the advent of factory fish farms that produce fish faster, fatter, and cheaper. Aquaculture is imitating agriculture. These fish are fed concentrated fish meal laden with both antibiotics to reduce disease and an unintended ingredient—polychlorinated biphenyl (PCB). The latter is a proven cancer-causing dioxin-like chemical banned in the United States in 1976 and slated by the United Nations for global phaseout.

Several studies from the United States, Canada, Ireland, and the United Kingdom have concluded that consumers worldwide are being exposed to elevated PCBs by eating farmed salmon. In 2003 the Environmental Working Group found that farmed salmon from five countries had sixteen times more PCBs than wild salmon, and four times more than in beef. A January 2004 study published in the journal *Science* found that farmed salmon had an average of 36.63 parts per million (ppm), while wild salmon had only 4.75.

Although these numbers are well below the allowable limits set by the U.S. Food and Drug Administration, which regulates fish sales, the agency's standards are seriously flawed. It has not updated its standards in twenty years, ignoring numerous peer-reviewed studies published since 1984. Even its sister agency, the U.S. Environmental Protection Agency, which regulates sportfishing, has limits 500 times more protective than those of the FDA.

By the way, farmed salmon don't turn out pink like wild salmon; they are pale yellow or khaki. Artificial color is added to the feed to redden them up. Look for the label with the words SUSTAINABLE WILD HARVESTED. It identifies fish that are "naturally grown." These fish are certified as organic by Farm Verified Organic, an organization with standards just as stringent for seafood procurement as the organic industry has for crop production. This label is currently your only guarantee that you are buying naturally cultivated, unadulterated fish.

Genetically Modified Foods

Imagine a world where pesticides were no longer needed, where hunger was eradicated, and where our foods provided pharmaceutical benefits. This is the promise of genetic engineering (GE) in agriculture, also known as biotechnology (BT) crops. In this plan, we are creating genetically modified organisms (GMOs) by taking the DNA from, say, bacteria, viruses, fish, or insects and adding them to another species, such as corn or rice. Thus, if we insert the gene of a pest-eating bacteria into corn, the corn would theoretically no longer need outside pesticides to fight off the bugs. It would literally carry its own built-in pesticide. Proponents of genetic engineering claim it is an extension of crossbreeding. Why shouldn't we, they say, produce wheat with the vitamin A gene from carrots if it can prevent blindness in the undernourished?

> **We simply do not know the long-term consequences for human health and the wider environment, of releasing plants bred in this way. . . . Do we have the right to experiment with, and commercialize, the building blocks of life?**
>
> —Prince Charles of England

Opponents say GE foods are morally wrong. They feel it is ethically abhorrent to cross the DNA of a fish, for example, with a vegetable. Scientists and experts can see both sides of this issue. Many do not want to impede progress, especially when it may be for the betterment of humankind. But there are problems. Doctors are concerned that new proteins will create new allergies. The U.N. Food and Agriculture Organization (FAO) blames hunger not on food shortage but on distribution problems exacerbated by poverty, politics, and the misallocation of resources.[12] Scientists from the Pesticides Action Network argue that genetically engineered soybeans don't reduce pesticide use at all but actually increase it.[13] USDA statistics from 1997 showed a 72 percent increase in the use of the popular herbicide glyphosate (brand name Roundup) resulting from the expanded use of the genetically engineered Roundup Ready soybean, which is designed to eliminate herbicides.

Commercialize is a key word in this controversy. After all, GE foods are brought to you by the same folks who make pesticides. Since the 1970s a large number of patents for seeds have been granted to petrochemical corporations. Critics worry about the concentration of power in a handful of chemical-food giants. GE companies are already demanding royalties on their seeds, even from farmers who never actually grew them! How can this be? The GE companies' argument is: If you are a corn farmer, organic or conventional, and the corn you planted is "contaminated" by spores from GE corn blown over from an adjacent field, which will make your corn grow as if it were GE corn, you must pay the GE company for use, intentional or not, of its seed. Will Mexicans one day be forced to pay royalties to plant maize, a crop they pioneered centuries ago? These are troubling issues that the courts are presently struggling with.

One of the most disconcerting issues about GMOs is that presently there are no regulations or labeling laws to identify them. This situation is compounded by the fact that 80 percent of the products in U.S. supermarkets contain some GMOs.[14] Soy, corn, potatoes, tomatoes, canola, cotton, papayas, radicchio, and squash are the main crops subject to genetic tweaking, and soy and corn derivatives end up in most processed (boxed or canned) foods. In a 2003 USDA-funded survey, 94 percent of Americans said they wanted their GE foods labeled. Forty-five percent of people responding to a 2001 Pew Initiative on Technology survey declared they were not confident the government could ensure their safety when it comes to GE foods. Presently neither the chemical companies nor the government regulators provide sufficient security for those of us (vegetarian people and animals) on the bottom of the food chain. The only way to safely avoid GE foods is to buy certified organic.

> **In my office I have tested hybrid and GMO foods versus heirloom and organic grains and some people will get symptoms of allergies from the new GMO grains and not from the older, natural ones. I am convinced that creating a new variant with different proteins and the adding of bacteria strains, etc. is basically creating a different food that is far more prone to causing allergies and compromising our immune systems in the long run.**
>
> —Dr. Lawrence Bronstein[15]

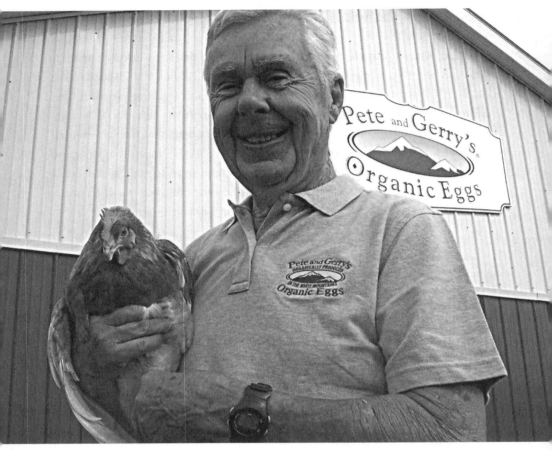

That's Grandpa Les Ward, former World War II Navy pilot who started his organic chicken farm with 5,000 uncaged chickens. Today he has 80,000 chickens. Sound like a lot? Not really! But the average conventional farm houses 5 million chickens in battery cages stacked twelve levels high.
COURTESY PETE AND GERRY'S ORGANIC EGGS

NUTrITION:

ARE ORGANIC FOODS MORE NUTRITIOUS?

One should eat to live, not live to eat.
—Molière, 1662

A re organic foods more nutritious? Yes! Although sometimes they may not look as pretty, gram for gram, organic foods rate higher in vitamins, minerals, and other nutritive plant compounds than conventional foods. And why not? A vegetable is only as good as the soil in which it is grown. Because organic vegetables are grown in rich, nutritious soil, they naturally contain higher amounts of minerals. In a study analyzed by the Australian Government Analytical Laboratory (AGAL), tomatoes, beans, peppers, and beets grown on organic farms, using natural soil-regenerative techniques, contained ten times more mineral content than the same foods grown by conventional means.[1] Since minerals are the building blocks of vitamins, the soil is one of the secrets behind the nutritional superiority of organic foods.

MORE VITAMINS AND MINERALS

There is mounting evidence that organically grown foods generate more nutrients and fewer nitrates. In a review of 400 published papers comparing organic and nonorganic foods, Soil Association Certification Ltd. of the United Kingdom reported that organic crops were higher in essential minerals, phytonutrients, and vitamin C.[2] Phytonutrients are plant compounds other than vitamins and minerals (such as enzymes, antioxidants, bioflavonoids).

In a 2002 University of Missouri study, chemists were shocked to discover that the smaller organically grown oranges delivered 30 percent more vitamin

C than the larger conventionally grown ones. Certified nutritionist Virginia Worthington found that a serving of organic lettuce, spinach, carrots, potatoes, and cabbage provided the recommended daily intake of vitamin C. But not so for the same veggies grown by conventional farming. Worthington reported that organically grown fruits and vegetables outpaced their conventional counterparts with as much as 27 percent more vitamin C, 21.1 percent more iron, 29.3 percent more magnesium, 13.6 percent more phosphorus, and 18 percent more polyphenols. Polyphenols are a group of plant compounds such as bioflavonoids, flavanols, and pycnogenols. They are anti-inflammatory and have a wide range of health benefits, including protection against allergies, arthritis, heart disease, cancer and more. The organics also showed 15.1 percent fewer nitrates and heavy metals than the conventional foods.[3]

Nutritional Advantages of Organic Foods

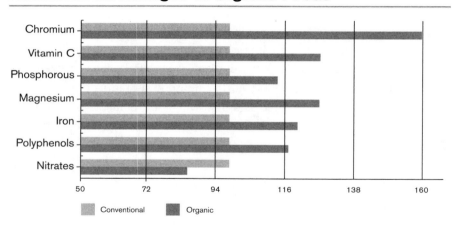

Organic foods are higher in key minerals and plant compounds and lower in unhealthy nitrates. See note 3.

Here's another interesting point. These phytonutrients, such as polyphenols and antioxidants, protect both people and plants. Pesticides—insecticides, herbicides, and fungicides—actually block a plant's ability to manufacture these important plant compounds. Without them, plants are handicapped and too weak to fight off pests. The organic farmer, on the other hand, builds up these important nutrients by feeding the soil, emboldening the plants to naturally defend themselves against pests and disease. In a study of antioxidants in organic and conventionally grown fruits, scientists found higher concentrations of valuable vitamin C, vitamin E, and other antioxidants in the organic foods. They theorized that the organically grown fruits developed more antioxidants as a defense and repair mechanism against insects when grown without the use of pesticides.[4]

Another important plant compound is salicylic acid. It is a major anti-inflammatory agent and among other things provides protection against rheumatism, hardening of the arteries, and colon cancer and reduces the death rate from heart attacks.[5] It was so useful that chemists synthesized part of it and called it aspirin! If you want the original version, eat organic vegetables. Biochemists at Dumfries and Galloway Royal Infirmary and at the University of Strathclyde in Scotland analyzed dozens of brands of organic and nonorganic soups and com-

> **Mothers are very critical organic consumers. They are very concerned with starting their babies off on the right track nutritionally. They know that organic foods offer pesticide-free nutrients that are also higher in antioxidants.**
>
> —Dr. Kathleen Delate, Iowa State University

pared their levels of salicylic acid. The organic soups had, on average, 600 percent more healthful salicylic acid than the other soups. The highest, an organic carrot and coriander soup, contained 1,040 nanograms of salicylic acid per gram compared with 20 nanograms in the average nonorganic soup.[6]

LOWER FAT IN MEATS

If you enjoy your meats but are concerned with higher quality with lower fat content, choose organic. The Swedish University of Agricultural Sciences studied thousands of cattle, sheep, and pigs and found that the organically raised animals had fewer health problems, better growth and fertility, and lower fat content than animals fed conventional feed.

Buy organic meats if you want to *steer* clear of "mad cow disease." You would be astonished at what they put in conventionally raised cattle feed: horse protein, tallow, blood products, pork remainders, poultry brain, spinal cord, and manure—quite an obnoxious diet, especially for a vegetarian animal that has been traditionally raised on grain and grasses! Cattle brain and spinal tissue were eliminated from U.S. feed in 1997 when they were suspected of causing mad cow disease (Bovine Spongiform Encephalopathy), a degenerative brain disease for cattle that has also been linked to a fatal human brain disease (Creutzfeldt-Jakob). The only beef in the United States that is free of this kind of feed and the potential it presents for mad cow disease is organic beef.

Could the extra pennies spent on organic foods possibly save us dollars later by helping us avoid the drugstore or the doctor's office? That is a ques-

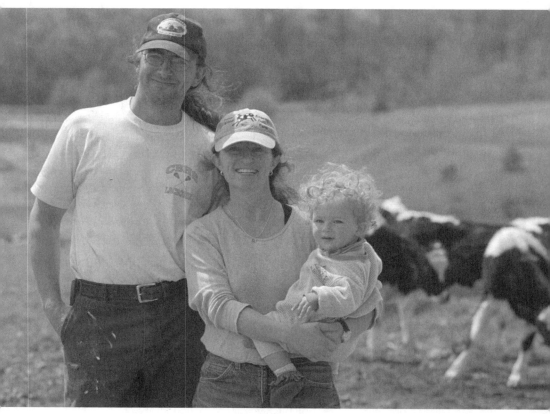

The Duetch family dairy farmers from Wisconsin believe it's never too early to start your children on organic foods. COURTESY ORGANIC VALLEY FAMILY OF FARMS

tion each of us must answer for ourselves, taking into consideration the health issues discussed in the previous chapter. But one thing is certain: You don't need a rocket scientist to tell you that organic foods are better for you. Yes, it's nice to see the research substantiating the extra nutrients in organic foods, but most of us never read science journals, and we certainly don't go shopping with them in hand!

We don't need a report to tell us that organic foods are more nutritious. If you think about it, nutrients don't come out of nowhere. They start in that soil enriched through composting, cover cropping, and humus. These organic techniques form the building blocks that make up the colors we see and the flavors we taste. Those vivid, vibrant colors and superior flavors are all the proof you need to understand how nutritious these foods really are. The proof is in the taste. *Taste*—now there's a mouthwatering subject that is worth exploring.

Taste:

DO ORGANIC FOODS REALLY TASTE BETTER?

There is no love sincerer than the love of food.
—George Bernard Shaw, 1903

Vitamins and minerals don't exist in a vacuum. It all starts with the soil. Rich soils create rich flavors. You can see the benefits of good soil in the colors and taste it in the flavors of these organic and natural foods. More nutrition means more flavor. We've just learned about the enhanced nutrition of organic foods. Well, more nutrients also means better taste.

FACTORS THAT AFFECT FLAVOR

Can you taste the difference between organic and nonorganic foods? In short, there are more "yes" answers to this question than "no"s. But this is not an easy subject for scientific evaluation. Let's face it, taste is a subjective matter. One person's caviar is another person's fish ovum! It is unlikely that any food can achieve a 100 percent consensus before a group of eaters.

In a 2003 tasting survey directed by the author, the organic foods tested were generally riper and juicier. Nevertheless, some tasters preferred the conventional foods because they were firmer and drier. The organic fruits were also generally sweeter, but some patrons preferred the tart conventional fruits. You can get any of these flavors from either organic or conventional fruits, but this is how they sorted out that day.

Okay, so we all have different preferences. But what about our proficiency as tasters? Are all taste buds created equal? No! It is an accepted fact that smoking dulls the sense of taste. Excessive salt in the diet and flavor stimulants

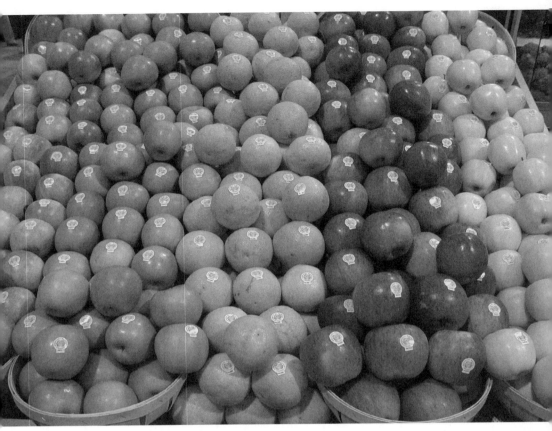

Organic fruits occasionally show blemishes. That is how naturally grown fruits look. Fungicides and insecticides may produce cosmetically perfect fruit. But organic fruits generally taste better.
STEVE MEYEROWITZ PHOTO

like MSG, along with the aging process, all contribute to a dulling of the taste buds. Taste is also dependent on the amount of moisture we produce in our salivary glands and even on how taste buds integrate with our sense of smell. By the way, husbands, don't even bother debating about the lasagna with your wife. Women have more taste buds than men do!

As if this were not complicated enough, agriculture introduces its own variables—season, location, soil, humidity, temperature, and degree of ripening before harvest. All these affect taste. So just because a fruit is grown using conventional methods does not preclude its potential for good taste. Organic bananas and carrots, for example, are famous for their superior taste. But on the day of our survey, the organic and conventional bananas and carrots available were similar in taste. However, when we switched brands of bananas, there was a clear difference in taste.

One other observation: People are willing to pay more for superior flavor. In our survey, the organic beefsteak tomato was $4.00 per pound and the conventional tomato was $2.00 per pound. The organic flavor was the clear favorite, and for those who favored it, the cost was not a deterrent, even at twice the price.

Organic Apples Are Sweeter

Scientists from Washington State University in Pullman rated organic apples the highest for sweetness, according to their tasting panels. Their comparisons included organic, conventional, and "naturally grown" fruits. The tasters labeled the organic apples sweetest, even after six months of storage![1] In a similar study by the Research Institute of Organic Agriculture (FiBL) in Switzerland, the organically grown apples achieved the highest scores in taste, sugar-acidity balance, firmness, and nutritional fiber content.[2]

Chimps Go Ape for Organic Bananas

If you want to do some serious banana tasting, ask the experts—monkeys! In an effort to become more ecological, the Copenhagen Zoo started feeding its animals some organic fruits. To their surprise, the chimpanzees were able to tell the difference between the organic and the regular fruit. In January 2003 zookeeper Niels Melchiorsen told the Danish magazine *Ecological Agriculture*: "For one reason or another, the tapirs and chimpanzees are choosing organically grown bananas over the others." It seems that they "instinctively tell the difference and their choice is not at all random." When the zookeepers left only the conventional bananas, the monkeys peeled them before eating. But they ate the organic bananas with the peel and all.

TASTE SURVEY: HOW IT WAS DONE

Our survey took the opinions of 175 people tasting sixteen items (eight foods). Most patrons tasted only two or three foods (four to six tastes). The survey was held at Guido's Fresh Marketplace, a large produce retailer selling both conventional and organic foods in western Massachusetts. All fruits and vegetables were matched according to their type so as to accurately compare, for example, a conventional Valencia orange with an organic Valencia orange.

Table 1: Author's Taste Survey

Food	Number of Tests	Favored Organic	Favored Conventional	No Difference
Plum	25	17	6	2
Banana 1	9	3	0	6
Banana 2	19	16	3	0
Orange	35	28	3	4
Tomato	34	26	5	3
Carrot	24	9	6	9
Cheese	29	18	11	0
Total	175	117	34	24

Source: Survey by Steve Meyerowitz at Guido's Fresh Marketplace in Great Barrington, Massachusetts, Summer 2003.

About half of the tastings were done as "blind" tastes, with the consumers not knowing which food they were tasting first. The majority of the patrons told us they rarely buy organic foods.

Table 1 describes the results. For example, you can see that out of 25 people who tasted plums, 17 preferred the flavor of organically grown plum, 6 preferred the conventionally grown plum, and 2 could not tell any difference. For the bananas, two brands were tested. On the first brand, 9 people tasted; 3 preferred the organic, none preferred the conventional, and 6 could not discern a difference. On the second brand, 19 people tasted; 16 preferred organic, 3 preferred non-organic, and none reported no difference. On this day, the most sensational foods were the oranges and tomatoes. Carrots, usually superior as organic, were not very competitive this day, nor was the organic cheese.

Despite its small size and informal nature, this survey clearly demonstrated that organic foods taste better. Out of 175 people, 117 preferred the organic foods, while only 31 favored the conventional and 24 tasters could not tell the difference.

> **We don't want to change the world, just breakfast, lunch, and dinner.**
>
> —Paul Wenner, author of *Garden Cuisine*.

price:

REAL COSTS AND VALUE OF ORGANIC FOODS

Nowadays people know the price of everything
and the value of nothing.

−Oscar Wilde, *The Picture of Dorian Gray*

Okay, it's true, organic foods often cost more. You don't need a book to tell you that! Typically, they cost approximately 25 percent more ($1.00 vs. $1.25), but there are plenty of examples of them costing both more and less than that. But to begin this discussion, we must ask: What are our shopping priorities?

WHAT KIND OF SHOPPER ARE YOU?

When we shop, we make our selections based on five basic criteria: *(1) price, (2) taste, (3) quality, (4) food safety,* and *(5) health and nutrition.* Is price your number one priority? Do you buy, for example, bruised fruit because of the reduced price? If price is your number one concern, then organic food is not for you.

Taste and quality are the next most important selection criteria. If you're like most people, you try to buy the best quality and flavor for your money. You must juggle taste, quality, and price. Ask yourself: Do you often buy the supermarket (store) brand?

If you are the parent of a young child, you have a choice of buying conventional milk containing bovine growth hormone (BGH) or spending more for organic milk that is BGH-free. The question becomes: What is the potential risk to your child's health?

- Price
- Taste
- Quality
- Food safety
- Health and nutrition

There is an endless list of qualitative decisions like these. But the first step is education. If you don't know about the health and safety issues surrounding BGH, for example, then your main criterion for buying milk will likely be price. Educating yourself about issues of health, food safety, nutrition, and organics is indeed . . . a good reason to buy this book!

Let's find out what kind of shopper you are. Ask yourself: When you go out to dinner, do you mostly eat at the chain restaurants? Do you always browse the menu according to price? Or are you sometimes willing to pay extra for perks like atmosphere? If you choose a relaxed dining experience and higher food quality, then price trails behind these considerations. If you are willing to spend money on atmosphere for restaurants, then you are a good candidate for spending the extra dollar, euro, or pound for organic food.

Another question: Do you ever buy gourmet food? If you are willing to spend the extra money for imported cheeses, gourmet chocolates, or preserves made by the local farmer, then you will be successful shopping for organic food. Organic is, in fact, a type of gourmet food. You might choose organic because it tastes better and is of higher quality. Again, taste and quality are competing against price. If these factors matter to you, then nutrition and health are not far behind.

Nutrition is a big subject. If you don't feel up to speed on nutrition, then here is a general principle that everyone can understand—*the better the quality, the better the nutrition.* So when you choose quality, you are already improving your nutrition. Another key principle of nutrition is freshness. The most nutritious foods in the supermarket are the fresh fruits and vegetables. The U.S. National Cancer Institute recommends five portions of fruits and vegetables every day as discussed on the Web site www.5aDay.com. Why? Because these foods hold within them nature's secret medicines. They're called phytochemicals—that is, plant compounds—including antioxidants, bioflavonoids, carotenes, enzymes, trace minerals, electrolytes, indoles, isoflavones, and glucosinolates. Here is another interesting fact. When fruits are attacked by insects, they produce more of these protective chemicals. So, if you notice a scar on your organic apple, don't get upset. That apple is healthier because it had to strengthen itself against attack, and you benefit from this extra nutritional reinforcement.

How do you measure the importance of health and food safety? In "Organic Foods: Healthier or Not?" we discussed the health advantages of organic food and some of the health and safety issues surrounding conventionally grown foods. The dangers of pesticides, antibiotics and hormones in livestock feed, and high-tech seeds impregnated with genetically modified organisms and artificial colors and flavors are all issues about which we need to be properly educated. The more we know, the safer the food choices we can make while shopping.

WHAT FACTORS SHAPE THE PRICE OF FOOD?

Now that you've got a basic understanding of the criteria involved in making a shopping decision, let's tackle the main subject: price. What factors shape the price of food? All foods, organic and conventional, are influenced by everything from the cost of trucking to labor, distribution, the price of oil in the Middle East

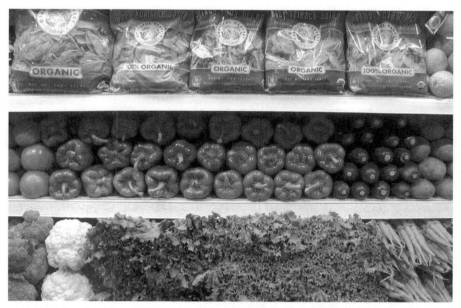

If an organic head of lettuce is $1.99 and conventional lettuce is $1.49, what is that fifty cents buying you? Is it peace of mind about bringing home safe, pesticide-free food for you and your family? Is it flavor and nutrition? STEVE MEYEROWITZ PHOTO

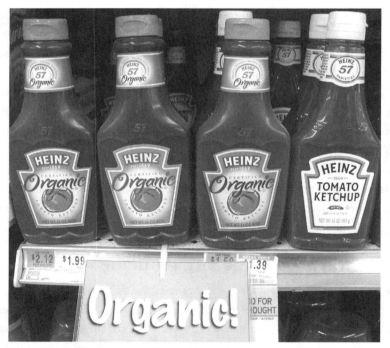

Heinz offers its organic ketchup (15 ounces) alongside its conventional ketchup (14 ounces). Yes, the organic ketchup costs more, but because its bottle is bigger, it's not as much more as you may think. STEVE MEYEROWITZ PHOTO

(for jet fuel), politics, subsidies, drought, and rain. Organic foods share these same expenses plus some additional ones.

Consider this: The popular Newman's Own brand of organic cookies used to include corn syrup bought from California. But because of cross-pollination from GMOs, the company must now import it from faraway Australia where GMOs are banned. The result: Certified organic cookies cost more.

And think about this: In 1956 Americans spent about 18.6 percent of their income on food. They spend about 9 percent today, according to USDA's Economic Research Service (ERS). But the farmer's share of each food dollar has dropped steadily, from forty-one cents in 1950 to only twenty cents in 1998. When you factor in inflation, this amount is so low that small farmers cannot survive. In 1997 the USDA reported that half of the U.S. farm production came from only 2 percent of its farms.

But it is market share and demand that have the greatest impact on prices. In 2003 organic foods sales represented only 2.5 percent of total U.S.

food sales and 3 to 4 percent of total European Union sales, according to the Research and Markets "Organic Foods Report." When you get to the bottom of the ledger sheet, it is this economy of scale that is the main factor working against the better pricing of organic foods. As you will see from the price comparison tables in this chapter, in spite of the industry's relative small size and extra costs, organic foods can be not only competitive but even less expensive.

Organic Prices: A Bright Future

Do organic foods always cost more? No! Just look at Table 3 (on page 65) to see how many organic bargains there are. Major supermarket chains are jumping on the organic bandwagon. They are opening up organic departments and discounting them with their own brand names. Why? Because demand for organics is increasing worldwide. According to the U.S. Department of Agriculture (USDA), U.S. organic food sales, approximately $11 million in 2003, have been expanding by an impressive 20 percent growth rate every year since the early 1990s. Imagine if your bank account grew at that rate!

Europe's organic industry is equal in size to the United States, but its shoppers are even more committed. You can tell just by walking into one of their McDonald's. McDonald's restaurants in Europe sell organic milk. Organic dairy in Europe has gone mainstream. According to the International Federation of Organic Agriculture Movements (IFOAM), Denmark's sales of organic milk jumped to 22 percent of total milk sales in the aftermath of the 2001 mad cow disease crisis. In Italy organic baby food products outsell conventional baby foods. In Switzerland the government invested 10 million Swiss francs, and Germany invested over 20 million euros to promote their respective organic food industries. Driving through Germany you can't help but notice organic products being promoted in magazines, on billboards, and on TV. One of the country's leading supermarket chains, Edeka, claims that its Bio-Wertkost brand (literally, "organic value food") represents 10 percent of its total sales. It doesn't stop in Europe. In Egypt, a tea-drinking country, the number one best-selling tea is a certified organic brand.

Organic is no longer a niche market, and its popularity is not just a fad. It represents a steady, permanent growth driven by the demand of shoppers demonstrating their willingness to pay for the benefits of flavor, quality, health, nutrition, and food safety. Price is secondary. More and more consumers recognize that the healthiest way to produce food is by organic farming. Although there is not a fair competition with conventional farming yet, market share is increasing, and the bigger it gets, the more prices are going to come down.

HOW TO GET THE BEST PRICES

In addition to national economics and the ups and downs of production costs, you will notice numerous price fluctuations at the local level. The best thing you can do to save money is to get to know your local stores. Visit the supermarkets, produce merchants, farm stands, and farmers' markets and compare prices on your favorite items. Prices, especially for produce, fluctuate locally from store to store, week to week, and season to season, but the best deals come from specials and sales. Watch for sales! Look in the newspapers, read the store handouts, and scan for the little sale signs on the shelves.

As you walk the aisles, be a detective. Some markets intermingle organic and nonorganic products; other stores segregate them. It is harder to comparison shop if the organic products are displayed separately. If they are intermingled, it

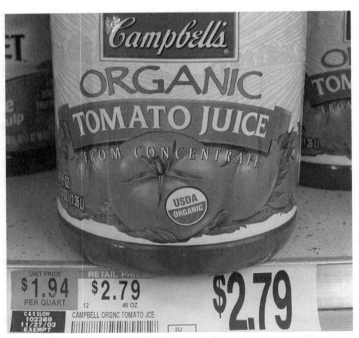

Do you need help reading the shelf tags at your supermarket? The unit price of this tomato juice is $1.94. In this case, a "unit" is a quart or 32 ounces. The product is 46 ounces and costs $2.79. Be sure to look for the USDA organic seal as well as the word "Organic" on the label. STEVE MEYEROWITZ PHOTO may also be difficult to find them because they get lost in the larger sea of conventional products. Look for signs or shelf talkers—small signs on the shelf edges. They announce the location of organic products and sales.

Carry your calculator! Different sizes of products make prices hard to compare. Look for unit pricing on the shelf tags to find the best bargains. But wait—they are not always there! For example, we found bags of baby spinach. The organic brand was tagged $4.99, and the nonorganic bag next to it was $2.99. Both bags looked about the same size, but they were not, and there was no unit price tag to be found! The *perceived* value favored the conventional brand, but the calculator revealed that the price per pound for the organic brand was actually $1.00 less!

Buy larger sizes whenever possible. It lowers your price per pound. Muir Glen's organic ketchup in the large 24-ounce size ($2.46/lb), for example, costs less than Westbrae's 13-ounce nonorganic ketchup ($3.18/lb). Bulk buying saves money. For fresh produce join a community-supported farm (see the CSA section in the first chapter) or an organic food co-op. For packaged foods join with friends to form a buying club. Buy by the case and save. The savings add up, and at the same time, you will make friends with like-minded shoppers.

How to Save $$ by Shopping Organic

- Look for sales. Read shelf talkers and store flyers. In some cases, organics cost less than conventional.
- Look closely. Many stores intentionally price organic items competitively.
- Carry a calculator. Read unit prices.
- Explore farmers' markets, natural food stores, and supermarkets and compare prices from store to store.
- Buy larger sizes. The price per unit drops dramatically when you buy a bigger jar, bag, or box.
- Buy in bulk and save. Join a club: a food co-op, buying club, warehouse club, or CSA farm.
- Buy locally and in season.
- Look for store brands or private-label brands.
- Choose a food you consume often and make a commitment to purchase it organically grown.
- Start your own organic garden.

Store Brands: Affordable Organics

Look for "organic" store brands. Store brands are privately labeled products produced for supermarkets by unidentified manufacturers. The store spares the costs of fancy packaging, advertising, and promotion and gets to have its own name on the product. The store makes extra margins (profits) by selling these products and passes the savings on to you. The consumer forgoes the comfort and quality assurance of brand-name recognition but gets a discount price. Sometimes the store name is not used, but other names such as Shurfine, Food Club, or Top Crest are used. These are private-label companies that buy from various manufacturers, put on their label, and sell to supermarkets. Because of their popularity, supermarkets are starting to develop their own private-label lines of organic products. This is good for them because

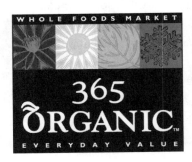

organics provide respectability and the impression of quality, something conventional private labels lack. It's also good for shoppers, since it reduces prices and increases the availability of organic products.

Whole Foods Market, the largest natural foods supermarket chain in North America, is telling its customers that they no longer have to pay premium prices for organics. Their 365 Organic brand label means organic foods are value-priced 365 days per year. Safeway Stores is a large U.S. supermarket chain with its own organic private label called Safeway Select Organic. Safeway supermarkets carry hundreds of items and intermingle the organics with mainstream products. Bargains are to be expected. Their Select Organic Raisin Bran Flakes, for example, sold for $3.59 per box the day we visited, and Safeway cardholders saved even more at a price of two for $5.00. Loblaws, the Canadian retail giant, has made organics mainstream with organic pasta sauce, tea, cheese, cookies, cake mixes, butter, English muffins, beef burgers, and even garden seeds under its President's Choice Organic brand. The chain's motto is: "Why pay over-the-top prices for natural goodness?" Kroger, the largest U.S. supermarket chain, has its Naturally Preferred line. Fresh Brands carries 850 natural and organic items under its Piggly Wiggly Naturals brand and proclaims: "Proud to Feature a Full Line of Organics." Full Circle is a private-label brand (see Tables 2 and 3) found in several supermarkets. It's by the same people who make Food Club, Top Care, Top Crest,

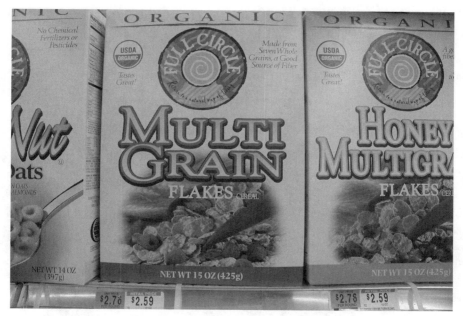

Private label brands such as Full Circle are helping to reduce prices and contribute to the rapid expansion of organic foods in supermarkets. STEVE MEYEROWITZ PHOTO

and Shurfine. Now they are going organic with hundreds of USDA-certified organic items that span every supermarket aisle. As reported in the trade journal *Private Label Magazine,* Full Circle says it created the new line to fulfill a desire by consumers who "recognize the relationship between diet and health" and "have concerns about pesticides." Private labels represent a milestone in the way organic products are marketed, and they mean lower prices for you.

About the Tables

If you think you can't afford organics, then take a look at the three tables in this chapter. You will be surprised. These prices were collected in typical super-markets. In this case, they were Price Chopper, the Big Y, and the produce market Guido's Fresh Marketplace, all located in western Massachusetts. The survey was taken in late summer of 2003. By the time you read this, organic products will be even more competitive, because as time goes on, the organic marketplace is growing, economies of scale are improving, and the increased competition is driving prices down.

Every effort was made to find comparable brands, with similar sizes and

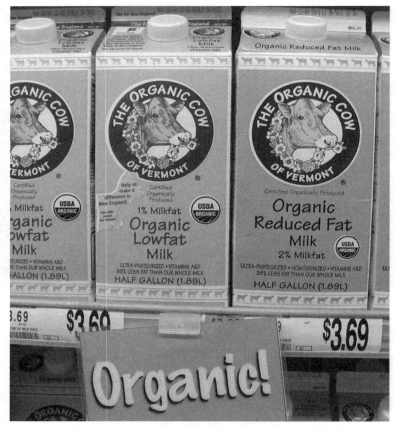

Shelf talkers are small signs on the edges of shelves in your supermarket that make it easy to locate organic items in a sea of conventional products. STEVE MEYEROWITZ PHOTO

packaging. Comparing a glass jar with a plastic jar, for example, would be unfair. Likewise, comparing a gourmet brand against a store brand would not be fair. Basically, we did not compare a high-end product against a low-end product. When shopping for tomato juice, for example (Table 3), RW Knudsen organic brand was compared to its own nonorganic brand. That's fair. We learned that Knudsen's charges only 10 cents more for its organic juice! But to compare this health brand to a store brand, for example, would not be fair. Same thing with orange juice. Organic orange juice is 100 percent pure squeezed, not made from concentrate, so you can't compare it with a mass-market producer of juice made from concentrate. Odwalla, a gourmet brand of freshly squeezed nonorganic orange juice, was $5.49 for a half gallon, and

Table 1

Price Comparison: Fruits and Vegetables–Organic vs. Conventional Foods
Prices in U.S. Dollars

Food	PRICE		BRANDS COMPARED	
	Organic	Conventional	Organic	Conventional
Banana	0.89	0.69	Per 16 oz.	Per 16 oz.
Grapefruit	1.59	0.96	each	each
Apples	1.99	1.39	Red delicious 16 oz.	Red delicious 16 oz.
Strawberries	5.99	4.99	Driscoll 16 oz.	Driscoll 16 oz.
Tomatoes	3.99	2.99	Per 16 oz.	Per 16 oz.
Celery	2.99	2.49	Per bunch	Per bunch
Carrots	0.99	0.59	Per 16 oz.	Per 16 oz.
Baby Carrots	1.79	1.49	Earthbound pkg./lb.	Baby Peeled pkg./lb.
Broccoli	1.79	1.59	Per 16 oz.	Per 16 oz.
Potatoes	1.39	0.79	Yukon 16 oz.	Yukon 16 oz.
Cabbage	0.99	0.59	Per head	Per head
Romaine Lettuce	2.29	1.29	Per head	Per head
Iceberg Lettuce	1.79	1.59	Per head	Per head

Source: Comparisons collected at Big Y and Price Chopper Supermarkets and Guido's Fresh Market-place in Massachusetts, Summer 2003.

organic by Horizon was $5.99 (Table 2). Full Circle brand organic is regularly $3.99 per half-gallon container; that's only 50 cents more than Tropicana's nonorganic, not made from concentrate, "premium" orange juice. But on the day of our survey, Full Circle was on sale for $2.99, making it 50 cents lower than the nonorganic Tropicana (Table 3).

When shopping for baby food, we compared Gerber's organic brand (called Tender Harvest) to its regular brand (Table 2). That's fair. Then we compared Gerber's Tender Harvest to Beech-Nut's DHA (Table 3). DHA is Beech-Nut's nutrition line. Both lines offer a little something extra, so they make a good match. (This is the reason why the World Boxing Association never puts a light-weight fighter in the same ring with a heavyweight!) Gerber's organic Tender Harvest brand had a lower price than Beech-Nut's nonorganic, DHA brand.

In the charts, when you see "/lb." or the word *per,* such as "per lb.," "per

Table 2

Price Comparison: Mostly Packaged Foods–Organic vs. Conventional Foods
Prices in U.S. Dollars

Food	PRICE		BRANDS COMPARED	
	Organic	Conventional	Organic	Conventional
Milk	3.49	2.89	Organic Valley 64 oz.	High Lawn Farm 64 oz.
Baby Food	0.67	0.55	Gerber Tender Harvest	Gerber regular
Yogurt	2.99	2.79	Stonyfield 32 oz.	Dannon 32 oz.
Soup	2.53	1.77	Amy's 16 oz.	Campbell's 16 oz.
Potato Chips	2.79	2.09	Kettle Chips 5 oz.	Kettle Chips 5 oz.
Peanut Butter	3.69	2.39	Store Brand 16 oz.	Store Brand 16 oz.
Salsa	3.79	3.59	Muir Glen 16 oz.	Newman's Own 16 oz.
Yellow Corn Chips	2.99	1.99	Tostitos 9 oz.	Tostitos Gold 9 oz.
Orange Juice	5.89	5.49	Organic Valley 64 oz.	Odwalla 64 oz.
Cranberry Cocktail	2.25	2.00	Full Circle per qt.	Ocean Spray per qt.
Ketchup	2.33	1.82	Heinz per lb.	Heinz per lb.
Corn Flakes	4.83	3.72	Natures Path per lb.	Kellogg's per lb.
Corn Flakes bulk	3.32	2.66	Natures Path bulk/lb.	Kellogg's bulk/lb.
Almonds	6.99	4.49	Raw almonds 16 oz.	Raw almonds 16 oz.
Cottage Cheese	3.99	1.99	Horizon 16 oz.	Head 16 oz.
Rice	2.09	1.59	White basmati 16 oz.	White basmati 16 oz.

Source: Comparisons collected at Big Y and Price Chopper Supermarkets and Guido's Fresh Market-place in Massachusetts, Summer 2003.

oz.," this means that the unit price is being presented. This was done in situa-tions where the product sizes were close but not identical. When unit pricing is used, comparisons were made with similar size products, since there are savings for buying larger sizes. It would be unfair, for example, to compare the unit price of a gallon of milk with a quart of milk.

Only a few prices listed in the tables are sale prices. Sales and specials are always ongoing. Thus, if an item was on sale during the survey, we included it as a valid price. But we did not include any closeouts or bruised produce prices. For example, we found a two-pound package of grapes by the Earth-

Table 3

Lower or Similar Prices for Organic Foods
Prices in U.S. Dollars

Food	PRICE Organic	PRICE Conventional	BRANDS COMPARED Organic	BRANDS COMPARED Conventional
Kale	1.49	1.79	Per head	Per head
Cauliflower	2.99	2.99	Produce, each	Produce, each
Romaine Lettuce	2.99	3.49	Earthbound pkg. of 3	Andy Boy pkg. of 3
Baby Spinach	4.99	5.98	Earthbound pkg./lb.	Fresh Express pkg./lb.
Kiwi Fruit	1.99	2.49	Earthbound pkg./lb.	Bulk Produce/lb.
Blueberries	4.99	4.99	Organic	Locally grown
Strawberry Jam	2.39	3.49	Sorrel Ridge 10 oz.	St. Dalfour 10 oz.
Applesauce	1.15	1.18	Full Circle per lb.	Mott's per lb.
Cantaloupe	3.99	3.99	Produce	Produce
Packaged Grapes	5.49	5.99	Earthbound 2 lb.	Grapes Under Glass 2 lb.
Apple Juice	2.49	2.69	After the Fall 32 oz.	After the Fall 32 oz.
Tomato Juice	3.39	3.29	RW Knudsen 32 oz.	RW Knudsen 32 oz.
Orange Juice	2.99	3.49	Full Circle 64 oz.	Tropicana Premium 64 oz.
Coffee	6.99	7.49	Java Love 12 oz.	Starbucks 12 oz.
Salsa	2.19	4.19	Enrico's 16 oz.	Desert Pepper 16 oz.
Salsa	2.99	3.99	Tostitos 16 oz.	Green Mtn. Gringo 16 oz.
Mustard	2.89	3.19	Eden, Dijon 8 oz.	Grey Poupon, Dijon 8 oz.
Ketchup	2.33	3.18	Heinz per lb.	Westbrae per lb.
Pasta Sauce	2.89	3.89	Muir Glen 32 oz.	Newman's Own 32 oz.
Pasta Sauce	1.78	2.55	Enrico's 32 oz.	Napa Valley 32 oz.
Eggs	1.29	1.29	Feather Ridge/dozen	High Lawn/dozen
Baby Food	2.40	2.76	Gerber Tender Harvest/lb.	BeechNut DHA/lb.
Popcorn	2.39	2.99	Full Circle 9 oz.	Orville Red. 9 oz.

Source: Comparisons collected at Big Y and Price Chopper Supermarkets and Guido's Fresh Marketplace in Massachusetts, Summer 2003.

bound organic brand for $5.49. That beat out the $5.99 price for a similar two-pound package by the nonorganic gourmet brand Grapes Under Glass (Table 3). On the day of the survey, the $5.49 price was on sale for $2.99. Nevertheless, we used the regular price instead of the sale price in this instance because we decided it was a closeout price. (Either way, the organic was cheaper!)

There were several instances in which one company makes both organic and conventional lines. For example, Driscoll, the berry and fruit packager, sells organic strawberries for $5.99 and conventional strawberries for $4.99 (Table 1). RW Knudsen, Heinz, Gerber's, and After the Fall, to name a few, all sell both. This makes for excellent price comparisons since the same company has the same overhead and distribution expenses. After the Fall's organic apple juice, by the way, was actually twenty cents lower (Table 3) than its nonorganic juice!

WHY DO ORGANIC FOODS COST MORE?

Organic farmers don't spend all day in their field. They can't—they have too much paperwork! As you may remember, organic farmers have more regulations, more inspections, more labor, more management chores, and more distribution expenses than conventional farmers do. Inspections continue all the way through the distribution system to ensure that organic products do not mingle with conventional foods. You may see an example of this in your supermarket if you see organic apples prebagged. This practice prevents store employees from accidentally mixing the fruit. But that bagging represents extra labor and materials expenses. Now add to the payroll the laborers who hand-pick, weed, and prune to keep the crops healthy and free of disease. Organic puts the human face back on farming. It employs people and builds local economies, and that's good—but it's expensive. Because of all these extra costs, organic cannot be fairly compared with the price of conventional foods.

Getting Food to You

Distribution is a major expense. According to the Worldwatch Institute, our food travels on average 2,000 miles from field to dinner table. This means gasoline, trucks, airplanes, tires, maintenance, breakdowns . . . it adds up. Conventional foods can manage these costs better because they save money on volume. Organics represent only $12 billion of the total $485 billion U.S. food market, making their overhead costs significantly higher. That's according to the 2003

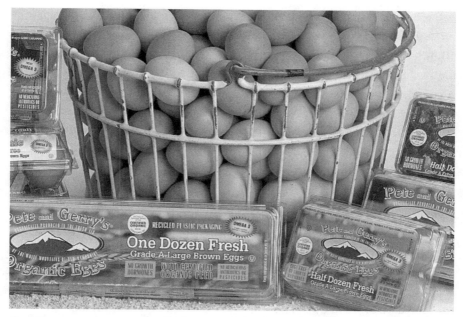

Eggs. No cages, no hormones, no antibiotics, no pesticides. Just organic feed and don't forget the recycled plastic packaging. COURTESY PETE AND GERRY'S ORGANIC EGGS

"Organic Foods Report" published by Research and Markets. Organic growers also have more intermediaries, shippers, and truckers and less of a financial cushion to buffer against a tough season.

Some Factors Affecting the Cost of Organic Foods

- More regulations; higher management costs
- More manual labor; bigger payrolls
- Smaller distribution; higher freight
- Picked ripe; no preservatives; shorter shelf life
- More research costs; no subsidies

Innovation Costs Money

As a farmer, if you're not going to use chemicals, all you have is your hands and your head. Organic farmers must spend money on education to learn the techniques of their trade. It was not until 2003 that the U.S. Department of Agriculture started to invest any government money for research, training, or development of organic farming. Instead, that burden has fallen on the individual farmer. Organic farmers must invent their own natural insecticides. They extract pyrethrum from chrysanthemums or squeeze the oil from the neem tree to create soapy sprays. They hang plastic owls in the trees to scare away berry-stealing birds. The costs of the research and training behind these techniques is hidden from consumers. Federal subsidies and tax abatements, common for conventional farmers, are almost nonexistent for organic farmers. It is not a level playing field. But this is slowly starting to change, and as it does, prices for organics will reduce to more competitive levels.

PRICE VS. VALUE

What value do we get from organic farming besides good food? Arguably, it is a sustainable future and a healthier ecosystem. Organic farmers work in harmony with nature. Every action they take protects the purity of our soil, water, and air for future generations. The soil is the foundation of the food chain. Organic farmers build the soil and protect it from erosion. They preserve seeds of special varieties; they protect wetlands, and through crop rotation, they provide foraging for wildlife. In short, organic farming minimizes the impact of agriculture on the environment.

Your investment in organic foods, the extra 50 cents or more, also contributes to a healthier economy. Organic foods are generally grown closer to home, meaning your money stays in your region longer, creates jobs, preserves seed varieties, and develops local cuisines. Far too many small farms in the United States have been sold and converted into strip malls and condominiums. A successful farm, on the other hand, keeps the land green for future generations.

SHOPPING POWER

As consumers we don't have the choice of what to stock on the supermarket shelves. We only have a choice of where to shop and what to buy. But always remember that these decisions influence the choices of food purchasing agents. If you want to see more organic foods available, keep buying them. Your selections affect not only your health and that of your family but also the public health. Organic foods are reflective of a larger movement of increased awareness about personal health and the environment. Organic farming was never designed to produce large volumes of food at low prices. It was designed to produce high-quality, nutritious food while respecting the health of people and animals. While conventional food stores ask "Will it sell?" organic food stores ask "Should it be sold?" As shoppers we vote with our food dollars, and ultimately our votes are either part of the solution or part of the problem.

> **Your food choices can be of tremendous benefit . . . the healthiest, tastiest, and most nourishing way to eat is also the most economical, most compassionate, and least polluting . . . You benefit, the rest of humankind benefits, the animals benefit, and so do the forest and the rivers and the soil and the air and the oceans.**
>
> –John Robbins, *Diet for a New America*, 1987

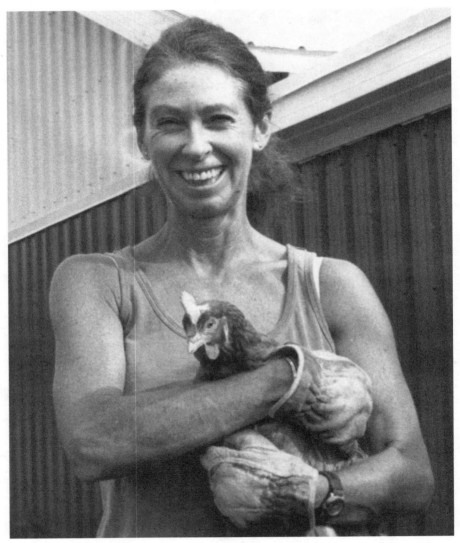

Carol LaFlamme nurses the chickens at Pete and Gerry's Organic Eggs in the Connecticut River Valley in New Hampshire. COURTESY PETE AND GERRY'S ORGANIC EGGS

HOW TO GET STARTED EATING ORGANIC

In five years, organics will be everywhere.
—Scott Van Winkle, market analyst, Adams, Harkness, & Hill, 2003

I t's safer, healthier, more nutritious; it tastes better, and prices are coming down. So what's not to like? Why not shop for organic foods right now?

There will come a day when you will find organic food served on airlines, in school cafeterias, at football games, and in convenience stores. You won't have to wait too long. The new Delta Air Lines subsidiary named Song has started serving organic food on some of its flights. Organic hamburgers have now replaced conventional burgers in all University of Wisconsin student cafeterias. Some football stadiums already offer vegetarian soy hot dogs, and 7-Eleven, the largest convenience chain store in the United States, has started stocking organic snacks.

Organic foods are in more markets now than ever before. Kroger, the number one supermarket chain in the United States, in 2003 was aggressively adding natural and organic food departments to over 1,135 of its stores. Its Naturally Preferred brand of premium-quality natural and organic products includes baby food, pastas, cereal, snacks, milk, and soy items. According to Kroger representative Gary Rhodes, "Natural and organic foods comprise one of the fastest-growing parts of our business." Even the staunchly conventional Wal-Mart, now the largest U.S. retailer of groceries, has started adding organic

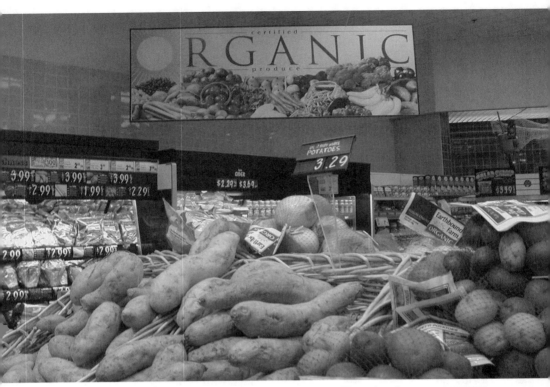

The organic department at a Price Chopper Supermarket in western Massachusetts. STEVE MEYEROWITZ PHOTO

foods to its Healthy Living section in some stores. Poultry industry leader Tyson Foods is distributing its Nature's Farm Organic Chicken in many supermarkets. At $5.99 a pound vs. the conventional no-name brand at $4.99 a pound, Tyson is betting consumers are willing to pay a little more for better quality. In 2002 Heinz began selling organic ketchup, and Frito-Lay introduced Tostitos Organic Tortilla Chips. Ben & Jerry's Homemade started testing organic versions of four of its popular ice cream flavors. True, the organic industry represented only 2.5 percent of the $485 billion U.S. food business in 2002, according to a 2003 *Nutrition Business Journal* report. But with retail sales growing at an average of 23 percent per year, organic foods were projected to double in size and achieve 4 percent of total U.S. sales by 2005. Convenience and availability are increasing; prices are decreasing. These food giants are betting on the future, and so should you.

How to Get Started

- Pick one food you like: milk, coffee, eggs, anything. Commit to always buying it organic.
- Taste test organic foods. Find ones that you like and add them to your repertoire.
- Explore the organic section in your local market. Try to find some new and interesting things there.
- Get to know organic drinks: sodas, milk, juice, or wine.
- Pledge to buy organic foods for your infant or child.
- Splurge on organic treats like chocolates, cookies, ice cream, lollipops, raisins.
- Bring some organic coffee beans to the office and share them with your coworkers.
- Visit a farmers' market and talk to the organic farmers.

Other Suggestions for Beginners

- Start an organic vegetable garden or try indoor gardening (sprouting seeds, such as alfalfa, without soil to use in salads or stir-fries). Share the bounty with friends.
- Create a party with an organic theme. Serve organic pizza, chips, salsa, cookies, tea, coffee, etc.
- Start a compost pile with your kitchen scraps.
- Buy a shirt or pillow made from organically grown fibers. (Studies show growing conventional cotton requires one pound of pesticides to produce three T-shirts.)

How do new shoppers get started? For many families the starting point is the arrival of their first child. New parents are learning about the dangers of pesticides and are convinced they need to serve their newborn safe, pure food. Studies such as the one done for Gerber and presented at the American Dietetic Association's annual conference in 2003 about "junk food babies"—infants and toddlers being fed soda, pretzels, and chips instead of fruits and vegetables—motivate new families to buy higher-quality foods. Organics fill that need.

Of course, another reason people start buying organic food is to improve their health. But for some it is not just about "health" but improving their overall feeling of "wellness"—a lifestyle change to achieve more energy, less stress, and good spirits. These people are moving away from foods like dairy products

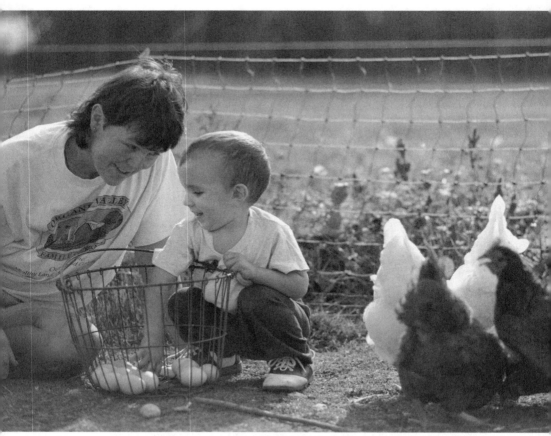

There's a lot of work in organic farming. But there are a great many happy moments too, as Gloria Varney of Maine and her family know. COURTESY ORGANIC VALLEY FAMILY OF FARMS

that cause allergies to act up and are instead buying alternatives such as soy milk and soy cheeses. Cholesterol-conscious folks are buying more meat substitutes and yogurts. This lifestyle shopping extends into products like organic pet foods, shampoos, and unbleached cotton sheets.

"Wellness shoppers" are not necessarily health purists. Even conventional shoppers' habits are evolving to include feeling good about where and how a product was made. More and more consumers are glad to know that their purchases are doing something good, whether it is helping the environment, local farmers, or farmers in the developing world. Call it "conscientious consumerism."

- More nutrition
- Great taste
- Competitive prices
- Reduced pesticide health risks
- No preservatives, artificial colors, or irradiation
- No genetically modified food
- Cleaner rivers and streams
- Purer drinking water
- More fertile soil. Less soil erosion
- Sustainable agriculture (farmland for future generations)
- Biodiversity—conserves plant and wildlife species
- Agricultural innovations
- Certification: A guarantee about how your food was produced

OUR SHOPPING POWER

Whether we realize it or not, we are part of the food chain. Soil creates plants; plants become food for animals; then plants and animals become food for people. Organic farmers are making new choices about how they treat soil and deal with the challenges of pests. Shoppers are also compelled to make new choices by considering the purity and quality of their foods. As consumers and producers continue to make better, more principled choices, the benefits ripple through the chain from soil to vegetable to planet to people.

For many years our society was convinced that cheaper food was better. But such is no longer the case. The residual costs of chemicals in agriculture are coming back to haunt us in the form of polluted air, water, and food—and ultimately higher taxes for the cost of cleanup and the effects on public and personal health. Unfortunately, it has taken us a few decades to learn that the cost of using chemicals in agriculture is more than just the price on the can.

Money is not the only capital of agriculture. Rivers, streams, forests, soil, air, water . . . they all belong to our natural capital. We need to value and protect these assets, too. How? By investing in them. What is the best investment vehicle? Our shopping cart. When we choose conventional, organic, GMO, all natural, fair trade, or whatever, we are investing not just in the end product—food—but in the entire sequence of events involved in the generation of that food. Don't think for a minute that your selections are too small to make a difference. On the plantations of South America, one farmer is called a peasant, but a thousand farmers are called a federation. Likewise, a thousand shoppers wield enormous authority, influencing decisions across a range of ecological, economic, and social issues. We are indeed the most powerful link in the food chain.

NOTES

How It All Began: Origins of Organic Agriculture

1. Verlyn Klinkenborg, "A Farming Revolution," *National Geographic Magazine* (December 1995).

Organic Foods: Healthier or Not?

1. Paul Lichtenstein, Niels V. Holm, and Pia K., "Environmental and Heritable Factors in the Causation of Cancer," *New England Journal of Medicine,* 343, no. 2 (July 2000).

2. Herbert L. Needleman and Philip J. Landrigan, *Raising Children Toxic Free* (New York: Avon Books, 1995).

3. Sheila Zahm and Aaron Blair, "Pesticides and Non–Hodgkin's Lymphoma," *Cancer Research,* 52 Suppl. (1992): S5485–88.

4. Michael C. R. Alavanja, et al., "Use of Agricultural Pesticides and Prostate Cancer Risk in the Agricultural Health Study Cohort," *American Journal of Epidemiology,* 147 (2003): 800–814.

5. C. Charlier et al., *Occupational and Environmental Medicine,* 60 (2003): 348–51.

6. Douglas L. Murray, *Cultivating Crisis: The Human Cost of Pesticides in Latin America* (Austin: University of Texas Press, 1994).

7. C. L. Curl et al., "Organo-phosphorus Pesticide Exposures of Urban and Suburban Pre-school Children with Organic and Conventional Diets," *Environmental Health Perspectives* 111 (2003): 377–82.

8. Commission on Life Sciences, National Research Council, *Scientific Frontiers in Developmental Toxicology and Risk Assessment* (Washington, D.C.: National Academies Press, 2000).

9. *Agricultural Pesticides: Management Improvements Needed to Further Promote Integrated Pest Management.* General Accounting Office GAO-01-815 (August 2001): 4.

10. Lisa A. Croen, Karen Todoroff, and Gary M. Shaw, "Maternal Exposure to Nitrate from Drinking Water," *Epidemiology,* 11, no. 3 (May 2001), 325–31.

11. Alex Trent, "Farm-Raised Salmon Linked to Contaminants," Salmon of the Americas media advisory (December 29, 2003).

12. Food and Agriculture Organization of the United Nations, Economic and Social Department, *Agriculture towards 2015/30,* Technical Interim Report (Rome: FAO, April 2000).

13. "Do Genetically Engineered Crops Reduce Pesticide Use? The Evidence Says Not Likely," World Wildlife Foundation—Canada media advisory (March 7, 2000).

14. Al Krebs, "New Poll—94% of Americans Want Labels on GE Foods," *Agribusiness Examiner #295,* www.ea1.com/CARP/ (October 19, 2003).

15. Dr. Lawrence Bronstein, DC, CNS, Diplomate of the American Clinical Board of Nutrition, certified BioSET™ allergy care practitioner. Mahaiwe Chiropractic and Holistic Services, www.mahaiwechiropractic.com (September 2003).

Nutrition: Are Organic Foods More Nutritious?

1. "Organic Produce More Nutritious than Conventional Says Australian Study," *Pesticides and You,* Beyond Pesticides/National Coalition Against the Misuse of Pesticides, 20, no. 1 (Spring 2000): 6.

2. Shane Heaton, "New Report Presents Evidence for Health Benefits of Organic Food," in *Organic Farming, Food Quality and Human Health* (Bristol, UK: Soil Association Press, October 2001).

3. Virginia Worthington, "Nutritional Quality of Organic versus Conventional Fruits, Vegetables, and Grains," *Journal of Alternative and Complementary Medicine,* 7, no. 2, (2001): 161–73.

4. M. Carbonaro et al., "Modulation of Antioxidant Compounds in Organic vs. Conventional Fruit (Peach, Prunus persica L., and Pear, Pyrus communis L.)," *Journal of Agriculture and Food Chemistry,* 50, no. 19 (September 11, 2001): 5458–62.

5. M. J. Eisenberg and E. J. Topol, "Pre-hospital Administration of Aspirin in Patients with Unstable Angina and Acute Myocardial Infarction," *Archives of Internal Medicine,* 156 (1996): 1506–10.

6. John Paterson, "Organic Food Might Reduce Heart Attacks," *New Scientist* (March 16, 2002): 10.

Taste: Do Organic Foods Really Taste Better?

1. John P. Reganold, et al., "Sustainability of Three Apple Production Systems," *Nature* 410 (April 2001), 926–30.

2. F. P. Weibel et al., "Are Organically Grown Apples Tastier and Healthier? A Comparative Field Study Using Conventional and Alternative Methods to Measure Fruit Quality," International Society for Horticultural Science *Acta Horticulturae* 517 (2000): 417–27.

resources:

CONSUMER ORGANIZATIONS

Consumers Union Guide to Environmental Labels, www.eco-labels.org. Developed by the publisher of *Consumer Reports.* Provides information on eco-labels, products, companies, and government standards.

Environmental Working Group, (202) 667–6982, fax (202) 232–2592; www.ewg.org. A not-for-profit environmental research organization. Much information and statistics on public health and the environment. Offices in Washington, D.C.

FoodNews.Org, www.foodnews.org. Point and click on different foods to learn what pesticides are used. Uses a large government-provided database. Produced by Environmental Working Group (EWG), above.

Local Harvest, www.localharvest.org. A public service project. Find farmers' markets, CSAs, food co-ops, etc.

Mothers of Organic (M.O.O.), (888) 444–MILK; www.moomom.com. Practical tips for protecting children from the dangers of poisons and pollutants in our food and environment.

National Campaign for Sustainable Agriculture, (845) 744–8448, fax (845) 744–8477; www.sustainableagriculture.net. Dedicated to educating the public on the importance of a sustainable food and agriculture system.

O'Mama Report, www.theOrganicReport.org. Online resource about organic agriculture and products, sponsored by the Organic Trade Association.

Organic Consumers Association, (218) 226–4164, fax (218) 353–7652; www.organicconsumers.org. A grassroots, nonprofit, educational organization representing consumers on food safety, environment, and agriculture.

Pesticide Action Network International, (415) 981–1771; www.pan-international.org. Ecologically sound alternatives to pesticides. Centers are worldwide.

PROFESSIONAL ORGANIZATIONS AND CERTIFYING AGENCIES

Biodynamic Farming & Gardening Association, (888) 516–7797, (541) 998–0105, fax (541) 998–0106; www.biodynamics.com. Nonprofit organization formed in 1938 to foster, guide, and safeguard the Biodynamic method of agriculture. Offices in Junction City, Oregon.

Certified Naturally Grown, (845) 256–0686; www.naturallygrown.org. Independent nonprofit that labels organic-like farms that are too small to participate in the national certification program.

Community Supported Agriculture, Robyn Van En Center for CSA Resources, Fulton Center for Sustainable Living, (717) 264–4141, fax (717) 264–1578; www.CSAcenter.org. The Robyn Van En Center offers a variety of services to existing and new CSA farmers and shareholders nationally.

Fair Trade Certified, www.transfairusa.org. About fair trade farms, products, and their certification program.

IPM Institute of North America, (608) 232–1528, fax (608) 232–1530; www.ipminstitute.org. International Pest Management standards, certification, and labeling. Educates farmers about how to reduce pesticide use; located in Madison, Wisconsin.

Organic Monitor, (44) 20–8567–0788, fax (44) 20–8567–0788; www.organicmonitor.com. The largest publisher of market research on the international organic food industry, located in London, England.

Organic Trade Association, (413) 774–7511, fax (413) 774–6432; www.OTA.com. Association for the organic industry in North America, located in Greenfield, Massachusetts. Excellent information resource.

INTERNATIONAL

Australian Certified Organic, www.bfa.com.au. The leading organic certifying agency in Australia.

Bio-Gro New Zealand, www.bio-gro.co.nz. The leading organic certifying agency in New Zealand.

California Certified Organic Farmers, www.ccof.org. The first organic certifying agency in North America.

Canadian Organic Growers, (613) 231–9047; www.cog.ca. Canadian informational network for organic farmers, gardeners, and consumers.

Demeter-International Certification Board, (49) 6155–8469–81, fax (49) 6155–8469–11; www.Demeter.net. International center for Biodynamic agriculture.

European Union, europa.eu.int/comm/agriculture/qual/organic. All about the EU organic program.

International Federation of Organic Agriculture Movements (IFOAM), www.ifoam.org. Nonprofit coordinator of the worldwide organic agriculture movement. Trade fair, magazine, conferences, directory.

Quality Assurance International, www.qai-inc.com. One of the leading organic certifiers with operations worldwide.

Soil Association Certification, www.soilassociation.org. The United Kingdom's leading campaigning and certification organization for organic food, farming, animals, and environment.

U.S. Department of Agriculture (USDA), www.ams.usda.gov/nop. Home of the U.S. National Organic Program (NOP).

PRODUCTS

Green Circle Organics, (540) 675–2627, fax (540) 675–1135; www.greencircle.com. Premier cuts from certified organic beef ranchers.

Johnny's Selected Seeds, (207) 861–3900; www.johnnyseeds.com. Organic gardening seeds.

Original Organic Company, (877) 874–3757; www.OriginalOrganic.com. Order organic and natural fruits and nuts for delivery to your door.

OrganicBouquet.com, (877) 899–2468; www.OrganicBouquet.com. Organic, pesticide-free online flowers.

OrganicKingdom.com, (877) 274–5914; www.organickingdom.com. More than 650 organic foods and health-related products.

Sproutman's Organic Sprouting Seeds, (800) 695–2241; www.Sproutman.com. Indoor gardening seeds and home sprouters.

Whole Foods Market, Inc., (512) 477–4455; www.wholefoods.com. World's largest retailer of natural and organic foods.

PUBLICATIONS

The Chemical-Free Lawn: The Newest Varieties and Techniques to Grow Lush, Hardy Grass, Warren Schultz, Rodale Press, 1989.

Living Organic: Easy Steps to an Organic Family Lifestyle, Adrienne Clarke, editor. Sourcebooks, Inc., 2001.

Organic Gardening Magazine. Rodale Press, www.organicgardening.com.

Organic Living: Simple Solutions for a Better Life, Lynda Brown, DK Publishing, 2001.

Rodale's All-New Encyclopedia of Organic Gardening: The Indispensable Resource for Every Gardener, Marshall Bradley, et al., Rodale Press, 1993.

InDex

M

mad cow disease, 47
Manual of Organic Standards, 6
McDonald's, 33, 40, 57
meat, 47, 71
methyl parathion, 39
Mexico, 27
milk, 53–54, 57
minerals and vitamins, 45–47
M&M-Mars, 33
Muir Glen, 33, 50
mustard labels, 22

N

National Academy of Sciences, 36, 38,
    39
natural food *versus* organic food, 7
naturally grown food, 6–8
Nearing, Helen, 31
Nearing, Scott, 31
Newman's Own organic cookies, 56
nitrates, 36, 39, 46
"no preservatives" label claim, 24
Northeast Organic Farming Association
    (NOFA), 17
nutrition, 45–48

O

Odwalla, 62
"100% natural ingredients" label claim, 23
orange juice, 62–63
oranges, 45–46, 52
Oregon Tilth, 17
Organic Crop Improvement Association
    (OCIA), 17
organic farming, 1–6
    advantages, 37
    defined, 2
    fungus and disease treatment, 4–5
    government support, 67–68
    insects and pests treatment, 3–4
    inspections, 6–7
    origins, 29–33
    philosophy, 2–3, 6
    record keeping, 2, 6–7
    soil treatment, 3
    standards, 2
    weed treatment, 6
organic food
    benefits, 75
    defined, 2
    eating, 71–75
    key points, 6
    versus natural food, 7

purchase motivations, 35
Organic Foods Production Act (1990),
    15–16
organic seal, 18
Organic Trade Association (OTA), 27, 32

P

packaged food price comparison, 64
PCB (polychlorinated biphenyl), 41
peaches and pesticides, 39
peanut butter labels, 20
penicillin, 40
PepsiCo, 33
pesticides
    and cancer, 38, 39
    in children's diets, 38–39
    costs of, 2–3
    Integrated Pest Management (IPM),
        11–12
    in modern agriculture, 35–36
    and public health, 38
    synthetic, 16
Pesticides Action Network, 42
pests, organic treatment of, 3–4
Pew Initiative on Technology, 43
phytonutrients, 45, 46–47, 54–55
Piggly Wiggly Naturals, 62
Pillsbury, 33
pizza labels, 21
plums, 52
pollution, chemical, 31–32
polychlorinated biphenyl (PCB), 41
polyphenols, 46
potatoes, 46
poultry, free-range claim, 25
predators, natural, 4, 37
price, 51, 53–69
    comparison tables, 61–66
    factors affecting, 55–57, 66–67
    future, 37–58
    getting best price, 58–59
    shopping power, 68–69
    shopping selection criteria, 53–55
    store brands, 60–62
    versus value, 68
Prodecoop cooperative, 12

Q

Quality Assurance International (QAI), 27

R

"rBGH-free" label claim, 24
Robbins, John, 29, 69
Rodale, J. I., 31

ABOUT THE AUTHOR

Steve Meyerowitz was nicknamed "Sproutman" in the 1970s because his New York City apartment was always packed with gardens of home-grown, organic baby vegetables. They were part of his lifetime fight against chronic allergies and asthma. After twenty years of disappointment with conventional medicine techniques, he became symptom-free through his personally designed program of diet, raw juices, and fasting. In 1980 he founded the Sprout House, a "no-cooking" school in New York City teaching the benefits of a "living foods," vegetarian diet.

Steve is a health crusader and author of nine other books, including *Power Juices Super Drinks, Wheatgrass Nature's Finest Medicine, Juice Fasting and Detoxification,* and *Food Combining and Digestion.* He has been featured on television on PBS, the Home Shopping Network, QVC, and TV Food Network; and he has written features in *Better Nutrition, Prevention, Organic Gardening,* and *House & Garden* magazines. His "home-sprouters," the Freshlife Automatic Sprouter and the Hemp Sprout Bag, used for indoor organic gardening, are sold worldwide. You can learn more about his books and gardening inventions at www.Sproutman.com.

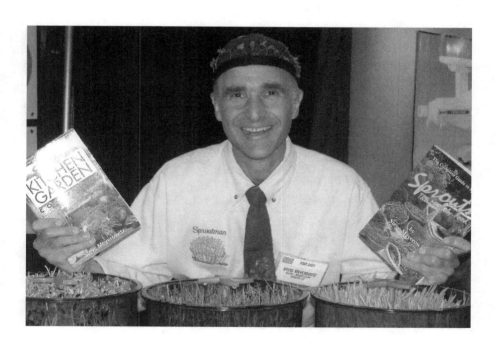

OTHER BOOKS BY STEVE MEYEROWITZ

WWW.SPROUTMAN.COM

Food Combining and Digestion
101 Ways to Improve Digestion

Water the Ultimate Cure
Discover Why Water is the Most Important Ingredient in Your Diet and Find Out Which Water is Right for You

Power Juices Super Drinks
Quick, Delicious Recipes to Reverse and Prevent Disease

Wheatgrass Nature's Finest Medicine
The Complete Guide to Using Grass Foods & Juices to Revitalize Your Health

Clinician's Complete Reference to Complementary/Alternative Medicine
Steve Meyerowitz, co-author. Edited by Donald W. Novey, M.D.

Juice Fasting & Detoxification
Use the Healing Power of Fresh Juice to Feel Young and Look Great

Sproutman's Kitchen Garden Cookbook
Sprout Breads, Cookies, Soups, Salads & 250 Other Low Fat, Dairy-Free Vegetarian Recipes

Sproutman's "Turn the Dial" Sprout Chart
A Field Guide to Growing and Eating Sprouts

Sprouts the Miracle Food
The Complete Guide to Sprouting